ISBN 0-8373-6125-7
25 CERTIFIED NURSE EXAMINATION SERIES

New **RUDMAN'S QUESTIONS AND ANSWERS ON THE...**

CN

Certified Nurse Registration Examination For...

Neonatal Intensive Care Nursing

Test Preparation Study Guide

Questions & Answers

NLC
NATIONAL LEARNING CORPORATION

National Learning Corporation

212 Michael Drive, Syosset, New York 11791

(516) 921-8888
(800) 645-6337
FAX: (516) 921-8743
www.passbooks.com
sales @ passbooks.com
info @ passbooks.com

PRINTED IN THE UNITED STATES OF AMERICA

PASSBOOK®

NOTICE

This book is *SOLELY* intended for, is sold *ONLY* to, and its use is *RESTRICTED* to *individual*, bona fide applicants or candidates who qualify by virtue of having seriously filed applications for appropriate license, certificate, professional and/or promotional advancement, higher school matriculation, scholarship, or other legitimate requirements of educational and/or governmental authorities.

This book is *NOT* intended for use, class instruction, tutoring, training, duplication, copying, reprinting, excerption, or adaptation, etc., by:

(1) Other Publishers
(2) Proprietors and/or Instructors of "Coaching" and/or Preparatory Courses
(3) Personnel and/or Training Divisions of commercial, industrial, and governmental organizations
(4) Schools, colleges, or universities and/or their departments and staffs, including teachers and other personnel
(5) Testing Agencies or Bureaus
(6) Study groups which seek by the purchase of a single volume to copy and/or duplicate and/or adapt this material for use by the group as a whole without having purchased individual volumes for each of the members of the group
(7) Et al.

Such persons would be in violation of appropriate Federal and State statutes.

PROVISION OF LICENSING AGREEMENTS. — Recognized educational commercial, industrial, and governmental institutions and organizations, and others legitimately engaged in educational pursuits, including training, testing, and measurement activities, may address a request for a licensing agreement to the copyright owners, who will determine whether, and under what conditions, including fees and charges, the materials in this book may be used by them. In other words, a licensing facility *exists* for the legitimate use of the material in this book on other than an individual basis. However, it is asseverated and affirmed here that the materials in this book *CANNOT* be used without the receipt of the express permission of such a licensing agreement from the Publishers.

NATIONAL LEARNING CORPORATION
212 Michael Drive
Syosset, New York 11791

Inquiries re licensing agreements should be addressed to:
The President
National Learning Corporation
212 Michael Drive
Syosset, New York 11791

PASSBOOK SERIES®

THE *PASSBOOK SERIES®* has been created to prepare applicants and candidates for the ultimate academic battlefield – the examination room.

At some time in our lives, each and every one of us may be required to take an examination – for validation, matriculation, admission, qualification, registration, certification, or licensure.

Based on the assumption that every applicant or candidate has met the basic formal educational standards, has taken the required number of courses, and read the necessary texts, the *PASSBOOK SERIES®* furnishes the one special preparation which may assure passing with confidence, instead of failing with insecurity. Examination questions – together with answers – are furnished as the basic vehicle for study so that the mysteries of the examination and its compounding difficulties may be eliminated or diminished by a sure method.

This book is meant to help you pass your examination provided that you qualify and are serious in your objective.

The entire field is reviewed through the huge store of content information which is succinctly presented through a provocative and challenging approach – the question-and-answer method.

A climate of success is established by furnishing the correct answers at the end of each test.

You soon learn to recognize types of questions, forms of questions, and patterns of questioning. You may even begin to anticipate expected outcomes.

You perceive that many questions are repeated or adapted so that you can gain acute insights, which may enable you to score many sure points.

You learn how to confront new questions, or types of questions, and to attack them confidently and work out the correct answers.

You note objectives and emphases, and recognize pitfalls and dangers, so that you may make positive educational adjustments.

Moreover, you are kept fully informed in relation to new concepts, methods, practices, and directions in the field.

You discover that you are actually taking the examination all the time: you are preparing for the examination by "taking" an examination, not by reading extraneous and/or supererogatory textbooks.

In short, this PASSBOOK®, used directedly, should be an important factor in helping you to pass your test.

CERTIFIED NURSE EXAMINATION SERIES

NURSING EXAMINATION RESOURCES

A variety of tests and programs are available through a number of organizations that will aid and help prepare candidates for nursing certification:

AMERICAN NURSES CREDENTIALING CENTER (ANCC)

The American Nurses Credentialing Center (ANCC) is a subsidiary of the American Nurses' Association (ANA), and the largest nursing credentialing organization in the United States. The ANCC Commission on Certification offers approximately 40 examinations including advanced practice specialties for nurse practitioners and clinical nurse specialists.

Certification is a most important way for you to show that you are among the best in your field – an extra step for you and your career, a step *beyond* state licensing. It gives you recognition and status on a *national* basis.

ANCC certification exams are offered twice a year in May and October in paper-and-pencil format, and throughout the year as computer-based exams. All exams are multiple choice and cover knowledge, understanding and application of professional nursing practice and theory. The time allotted for both the paper-and-pencil and computer certification exams is 3 hours and 30 minutes.

Each exam is developed in cooperation with an individual Content Expert Panel (CEP) composed of experts representing specific areas of certification. These panels analyze the professional skills and abilities required and then define which content should be covered and how strongly emphasized. Test questions are written by certified nurses in their discipline and reviewed by the ANCC to ensure validity and quality.

Exams are scored on a scale, and will be reported as either "Pass" or "Fail." Those who fail the exam will receive diagnostic information for each area of the test. There is a minimum 90-day waiting period from the date of the failed exam for those looking to retake it. For those who pass the exam, a certificate, official identification card and pin will be sent. Certification is valid for five years.

For further information and application for admission to candidacy for certification, write to:

American Nurses Credentialing Center
8515 Georgia Ave., Suite 400
Silver Spring, MD 20910-3492

You can also contact the ANCC and receive further details regarding certification exams and registration by visiting its home on the Internet – www.nursecredentialing.org – or by phone (1-800-284-CERT). Test Content Outlines (TCO) for each exam can also be found on the ANCC website, detailing the format and content breakdown of the test as well as the content areas the examinee should be prepared for.

NATIONAL CERTIFICATION CORPORATION

NCC CERTIFICATION

NCC – the National Certification Corporation for the Obstetric, Gynecologic and Neonatal Nursing specialties – is an independent certification organization. NCC was established in 1975 as a non-profit corporation for the purpose of sponsoring a volunteer certification program.

BENEFITS OF CERTIFICATION

Certification serves as an added credential to attest to attainment of special knowledge beyond the basic nursing degree. Certification serves to maintain and promote quality nursing care by providing a mechanism to nurses to demonstrate their special knowledge in a specific nursing area.

Promotion of quality care through certification benefits not only the individual nurse and the profession of nursing, but the public as well. Certification documents to employers, professional colleagues and health team members that special knowledge has been achieved, provides for expanded career opportunities and advancement within the specialty of OGN nursing, and elevates the standards of the obstetric, gynecologic and neonatal nursing practice.

Certification granted by NCC is pursuant to a voluntary procedure intended solely to test for special knowledge.

NCC does not purport to license, to confer a right or privilege upon, nor otherwise to define qualifications of any person for nursing practice.

The significance of certification in any jurisdiction or institution is the responsibility of the candidate to determine. The candidate should contact the appropriate state board of nursing or institution.

EXAMINATION DEVELOPMENT

NCC selects educators and practitioners in both nursing and medicine who possess expertise in the specialty areas within the obstetric, gynecologic and neonatal nursing and related fields to serve on the test committees. Responsibilities of the test committees include coordination of overall development of certification examinations and development of materials to assist candidates to assess readiness to participate in the certification process.

EXAMINATION DESCRIPTION

Each of the examinations consists of 200 multiple-choice questions. Two forms of each examination are often given to provide the opportunity to perform statistical procedures which ensure added reliability to the total examination process. The examinations are offered only in English and are designed to test special knowledge.

The examinations are given once each in the morning and afternoon, Monday through Friday, at more than 100 test centers. Four hours are allotted for completion of the examination.

THE CERTIFICATION PROCESS

1. Applicants must complete and file a certification application and appropriate documentation and fees
2. An acknowledgment postcard is sent to each applicant when NCC receives the application
3. Eligibility to participate is determined
4. Applicant is notified of eligibility status and eligible candidate receives a Candidate Guide to NCC Certification (4 to 6 weeks from receipt of application)
5. Candidates will schedule their own appointment for an examination time and location, and must take the exam within a 90-day period from notification of eligibility
6. Test administration occurs
7. Examinations are scored and analyzed
8. Candidates receive score reports upon completion of computerized testing (not paper testing)
9. Candidates are notified of certification status, receive information about certification maintenance and are later issued formal certificates

REVIEW COURSES AND NCC

NCC does not sponsor or endorse any review courses or materials for the certification examinations, because to do so would be a conflict of interest.

NCC is not affiliated with and does not provide input or information for any review courses or materials that other organizations may offer.

NCC views certification as an evaluative process. Eligibility criteria have been established to identify a minimum level of preparation for the exams.

CANDIDATE GUIDE TO NCC CERTIFICATION

Each candidate determined eligible to participate in the NCC certification process will be sent a Guide to NCC Certification. These guides can also be found online at the NCC website (www.nccnet.org). The Candidate Guides contain:

- General policies and procedures about the certification process
- Competency Statements that serve as a role description for the specialty nurse
- Expanded examination content outline
- Bibliography of references
- Sample questions to familiarize candidates with examination format (*These questions are not representative of exam content or difficulty level)

The Candidate Guide is not provided as study material, but to assist candidates in evaluating their own nursing practice as they prepare for the certification examination through identification of potential areas of strength and weakness.

SCORING OF EXAMINATIONS

Passing scores are determined based on a criterion-referenced system. Criterion passing scores are established by the NCC Board of Directors in conjunction with the NCC Test Committees using standard psychometric procedures.

Each question is statistically analyzed and evaluated with psychometric consultation, and scores are computed based on this evaluation.

Candidates who take the computerized form of the certification exam will receive their score reports upon completion of the exam. Those who take the paper/pencil exam will not receive their score reports for several weeks after administration.

NOTIFICATION AND AWARDING OF CERTIFICATION

Each candidate is notified of the success or failure to achieve certification. Successful candidates receive a formal certificate and will be able to use the initial RNC (Registered Nurse Certified) to indicate certification status.

Certification is awarded for a period of three years. Initial certification is effective from the date of notification to December 31 of the third full calendar year following notification. Subsequent periods of certification are subject to policies of the Certification Maintenance Program.

CERTIFICATION MAINTENANCE

The NCC Certification Maintenance Program allows the certified nurse to maintain NCC certification status.

Certification status must be maintained on an ongoing basis every three years through demonstration of approved continuing education or reexamination. Certification that is not maintained through the Certification Maintenance Program may only be regained by reexamination.

Specific information about the Certification Maintenance Program is provided to successful certification candidates and may also be obtained by contacting the NCC website (www.nccnet.org).

GENERAL POLICIES

All required practice experience/employment must have occurred while the applicant is/was a U.S. or Canadian RN. Graduate Nurse or Interim Permit status is acceptable, but must be indicated separately on the application form in addition to original licensure information.

NCC defines employment as practice in any of the following settings: direct patient care, educational institutions, administration or research.

When meeting educational requirements, all coursework, including that not directly related to specialty areas, thesis work and/or other program requirements must be completed at the time the application is filed.

It is the policy of NCC that no individual shall be excluded from the opportunity to participate in the NCC certification program on the basis of race, national origin, religion, sex, age or handicap.

All applications received are subject to the nonrefundable application fee ($250 paper/pencil; $300 computer).

Incomplete applications or applications submitted without appropriate fees will be returned and subject to all policies, fees and deadlines.

Applicants determined eligible (whether the candidate has been notified or not) and withdrawn will be subject to stated refund policies.

All NCC policies and requirements are subject to change without notice.

RETEST POLICIES

The NCC does not limit the number of times a candidate may retake the NCC Certification Examinations. Unsuccessful candidates who wish to be retested must reapply, submit all applicable fees and documentation, and re-establish eligibility.

Eligibility: All eligibility criteria of practice experience and/or educational preparation must be met by the time of application. It is the candidate's decision to choose the appropriate examination, based on the content outline, the individual's practice experience and NCC eligibility criteria.

Forms: All required forms must be submitted, and must include all requested information. If the forms are missing information, your application will be returned or you may be found ineligible to sit for the exam. Be sure the RN licensure information is completed. Be sure your documentation is signed by your supervisor or program director, with his/her title indicated, and the date the form is signed. Review your forms before you submit them.

Fees and Refunds: The proper fee must be submitted with your application or it will be returned.

For a current exam catalog containing current fees, terms, filing deadlines and exam dates, contact the NCC at www.nccnet.org, call (312) 951-0207 or fax at (312) 951-9475.

National Certification Corporation
PO Box 11082
Chicago, IL 60611-0082

CENTER FOR CERTIFICATION PREPARATION AND REVIEW

The Center for Certification Preparation and Review (CCPR) provides practice examinations developed by nurses and is intended to familiarize candidates with the content and feel of the real test. The CCPR practice examination identifies content areas of strength and weakness, provides examples of the type and format of questions that will appear on the examination, as well as information on how to focus additional study efforts.

The CCPR program consists of: study strategies, competency statements, content outline, 160-item examination, answer key and sample answer sheet, performance assessment grid, rationales for answers and cited references. Exams are available for inpatient obstetric, maternal newborn, neonatal intensive care and low-risk neonatal nursing, as well as neonatal nurse practitioner and women's health care nurse practitioner.

More information on ordering these practice exams can be found at www.ccprnet.org.

The National Certification Corporation (NCC), a not-for-profit organization that provides a national credentialing program for nurses, physicians and other licensed health care personnel, offers candidate guides for each of the NCC examinations. These candidate guides contain competency statements, detailed test outlines, sample questions, list of book/periodical references and all NCC policies related to the test administration process.

NCC guides are available in the following areas: inpatient obstetric, low-risk neonatal, maternal newborn and neonatal intensive care nursing, as well as neonatal nurse practitioner, telephone nursing practice, women's health care nurse practitioner, electronic fetal monitoring subspecialty examination, and menopause clinician. These guides, in addition to other information regarding testing, NCC publications and links to other organizations, are available online at www.nccnet.org.

RESOURCES FOR PRE-ADMISSION AND ACHIEVEMENT TESTS IN RN AND PN PROGRAMS

The National League for Nursing (NLN) offers a wide variety of examinations designed to aid students looking to further their education in the field of nursing. NLN pre-admission exams are reliable and valid predictors of student success in nursing programs, and NLN achievement tests allow educators to evaluate course or program objectives and to compare student performance to a national sample. The NLN also provides Diagnostic Readiness Tests, Critical Thinking and Comprehensive Nursing Achievement Exams and Acceleration Challenge Exams.

NLN exams can be ordered in paper form or e-mailed directly to you as online tests. The RN program includes tests in: basic nursing care, nursing care of children, maternity and child health nursing, nursing care of adults, psychiatric mental health and pharmacology in clinical nursing, baccalaureate achievement, physical assessment, community health nursing, comprehensive psychiatric nursing, heath and illness, anatomy and physiology, and microbiology.

NLN achievement tests also cover a PN program, which includes exams in: PN fundamentals, maternity infant, child health and adult health nursing, as well as mental health concepts and PN pharmacology.

NLN Pre-NCLEX Readiness Tests serve as practice and review for the NCLEX. Comprehensive Nursing Achievement, Critical Thinking and Diagnostic Readiness Tests are complementary to one another and help students prepare for nursing practice and to pass the NCLEX.

For in-depth information about the types of tests available, ordering, and additional NLN publications, including the NLN test catalog (available for download), visit www.nln.org.

NEONATAL INTENSIVE CARE NURSING EXAMINATION

CONTENT OUTLINE

Areas of knowledge to be tested on the NCC certification examination are listed below. This listing is not all-inclusive and is provided only to familiarize candidates with content that may be tested.

Percentages identified below represent a range of the number of test items assigned to each content area and therefore may total more than 100 percent. These ranges are based on the average percentages of examinations *previously* given and may not necessarily reflect current or future examinations.

HIGH RISK FACTORS (5-10%)
Antepartal
Intrapartal

GENERAL ASSESSMENT (10-15%)
Gestational Age (At Birth)
Physical Assessment
Baseline Laboratory (Knowledge and Interpretation)
Neurobehavioral Assessment
Community

GENERAL MANAGEMENT (25-35%)
Resuscitation and Stabilization
Fluids and Electrolytes
Nutrition and Feeding
Monitoring and Equipment
Oxygenation and Acid Base Homeostasis
Thermoregulation
Neonatal Hygiene
Pharmacology

ASSESS & MANAGE PATHOPHYSIOLOGIC STATES (30-40%)
Cardiac
Respiratory
GI (Gastrointestinal)
GU (Genital Urinary)
Integumentary
Musculoskeletal
Hematopoietic
Neurological
Infectious Diseases
Metabolic/Endocrine
Genetic Disorders
Head, Eyes, Ears, Nose and Throat

ASSESS & MANAGE PSYCHOSOCIAL/ BEHAVIORAL ADJUSTMENTS (5-10%)
Discharge Planning
Grieving Process
Family Integration
Infant Follow-up and Outcome
Promotion of Development

PROFESSIONAL ISSUES (5% or less)
Quality Assurance
Ethical/Legal Issues
Professional Relationships
Research Principles

HOW TO TAKE A TEST

You have studied long, hard and conscientiously.

With your official admission card in hand, and your heart pounding, you have been admitted to the examination room.

You note that there are several hundred other applicants in the examination room waiting to take the same test.

They all appear to be equally well prepared.

You know that nothing but your best effort will suffice. The "moment of truth" is at hand: you now have to demonstrate objectively, in writing, your knowledge of content and your understanding of subject matter.

You are fighting the most important battle of your life—to pass and/or score high on an examination which will determine your career and provide the economic basis for your livelihood.

What extra, special things should you know and should you do in taking the examination?

BEFORE THE TEST

YOUR PHYSICAL CONDITION IS IMPORTANT

If you are not well, you can't do your best work on tests. If you are half asleep, you can't do your best either. Here are some tips:

1) Get about the same amount of sleep you usually get. Don't stay up all night before the test, either partying or worrying—DON'T DO IT!
2) If you wear glasses, be sure to wear them when you go to take the test. This goes for hearing aids, too.
3) If you have any physical problems that may keep you from doing your best, be sure to tell the person giving the test. If you are sick or in poor health, you really cannot do your best on any test. You can always come back and take the test some other time.

AT THE TEST

EXAMINATION TECHNIQUES

1) Read the general instructions carefully. These are usually printed on the first page of the exam booklet. As a rule, these instructions refer to the timing of the examination; the fact that you should not start work until the signal and must stop work at a signal, etc. If there are any *special* instructions, such as a choice of questions to be answered, make sure that you note this instruction carefully.

2) When you are ready to start work on the examination, that is as soon as the signal has been given, read the instructions to each question booklet, underline any key words or phrases, such as *least*, *best*, *outline*, *describe* and the like. In this way you will tend to answer as requested rather than discover on reviewing your paper that you *listed without describing*, that you selected the *worst* choice rather than the *best* choice, etc.

3) If the examination is of the objective or multiple-choice type – that is, each question will also give a series of possible answers: A, B, C or D, and you are called upon to select the best answer and write the letter next to that answer on your answer paper – it is advisable to start answering each question in turn. There may be anywhere from 50 to 100 such questions in the three or four hours allotted and you can see how much time would be taken if you read through all the questions before beginning to answer any. Furthermore, if you come across a question or group of questions which you know would be difficult to answer, it would undoubtedly affect your handling of all the other questions.

4) If the examination is of the essay type and contains but a few questions, it is a moot point as to whether you should read all the questions before starting to answer any one. Of course, if you are given a choice – say five out of seven and the like – then it is essential to read all the questions so you can eliminate the two which are most difficult. If, however, you are asked to answer all the questions, there may be danger in trying to answer the easiest one first because you may find that you will spend too much time on it. The best technique is to answer the first question, then proceed to the second, etc.

5) Time your answers. Before the exam begins, write down the time it started, then add the time allowed for the examination and write down the time it must be completed, then divide the time available somewhat as follows:
    - If 3-1/2 hours are allowed, that would be 210 minutes. If you have 80 objective-type questions, that would be an average of 2-1/2 minutes per question. Allow yourself no more than 2 minutes per question, or a total of 160 minutes, which will permit about 50 minutes to review.
    - If for the time allotment of 210 minutes there are 7 essay questions to answer, that would average about 30 minutes a question. Give yourself only 25 minutes per question so that you have about 35 minutes to review.

6) The most important instruction is to *read each question* and make sure you know what is wanted. The second most important instruction is to *time yourself properly* so that you answer every question. The third most important instruction is to *answer every question.* Guess if you have to but include something for each question. Remember that you will receive no credit for a blank and will probably receive some credit if you write something in answer to an essay question. If you guess a letter – say "B" for a multiple-choice question – you may have guessed right. If you leave a blank as an answer to a multiple-choice question, the examiners may respect your

feelings but it will not add a point to your score. Some exams may penalize you for wrong answers, so in such cases *only*, you may not want to guess unless you have some basis for your answer.

7) Suggestions
   a. Objective-type questions
      1. Examine the question booklet for proper sequence of pages and questions
      2. Read all instructions carefully
      3. Skip any question which seems too difficult; return to it after all other questions have been answered
      4. Apportion your time properly; do not spend too much time on any single question or group of questions
      5. Note and underline key words – *all, most, fewest, least, best, worst, same, opposite,* etc.
      6. Pay particular attention to negatives
      7. Note unusual option, e.g., unduly long, short, complex, different or similar in content to the body of the question
      8. Observe the use of "hedging" words – *probably, may, most likely,* etc.
      9. Make sure that your answer is put next to the same number as the question
      10. Do not second-guess unless you have good reason to believe the second answer is definitely more correct
      11. Cross out original answer if you decide another answer is more accurate; do not erase until you are ready to hand your paper in
      12. Answer all questions; guess unless instructed otherwise
      13. Leave time for review

   b. Essay questions
      1. Read each question carefully
      2. Determine exactly what is wanted. Underline key words or phrases.
      3. Decide on outline or paragraph answer
      4. Include many different points and elements unless asked to develop any one or two points or elements
      5. Show impartiality by giving pros and cons unless directed to select one side only
      6. Make and write down any assumptions you find necessary to answer the questions
      7. Watch your English, grammar, punctuation and choice of words
      8. Time your answers; don't crowd material

8) Answering the essay question

Most essay questions can be answered by framing the specific response around several key words or ideas. Here are a few such key words or ideas:

M's: manpower, materials, methods, money, management
P's: purpose, program, policy, plan, procedure, practice, problems, pitfalls, personnel, public relations

a. Six basic steps in handling problems:
   1. Preliminary plan and background development
   2. Collect information, data and facts
   3. Analyze and interpret information, data and facts
   4. Analyze and develop solutions as well as make recommendations
   5. Prepare report and sell recommendations
   6. Install recommendations and follow up effectiveness

b. Pitfalls to avoid
   1. *Taking things for granted* – A statement of the situation does not necessarily imply that each of the elements is necessarily true; for example, a complaint may be invalid and biased so that all that can be taken for granted is that a complaint has been registered
   2. *Considering only one side of a situation* – Wherever possible, indicate several alternatives and then point out the reasons you selected the best one
   3. *Failing to indicate follow up* – Whenever your answer indicates action on your part, make certain that you will take proper follow-up action to see how successful your recommendations, procedures or actions turn out to be
   4. *Taking too long in answering any single question* – Remember to time your answers properly

EXAMINATION SECTION

EXAMINATION SECTION
TEST 1

DIRECTIONS: Each question or incomplete statement is followed by several suggested answers or completions. Select the one that BEST answers the question or completes the statement. *PRINT THE LETTER OF THE CORRECT ANSWER IN THE SPACE AT THE RIGHT.*

1. The assessment findings in the neonate with an imperforate anus do NOT include: 1.___
   A. Once the diagnosis of a low imperforate anus is made, a fistula should be sought
   B. In low lesions, there may be a thin membrane over the anal orifice, or there may be a fistula along the perineum and scrotal raphe
   C. If meconium passes in the urine or from the vagina, a high lesion is present
   D. In untreated patients, the subsequent intestinal obstruction will cause abdominal distention and constipation

2. All of the following are appropriate surgical interventions for the treatment of imperforate anus in the neonate EXCEPT: 2.___
   A. Preoperatively, the infant should be kept NPO and an orogastric tube should be placed. If a fistula is present on the perineum or fourchette, it should be dilated.
   B. After colostomy in infants with a high imperforate anus, a formal repair is undertaken at 16 to 22 months of age
   C. Approached via a posterior sacral incision, the blind ending rectum is brought through the sphincter mechanism and anastomosed to the anal skin
   D. After anoplasty, simple skin care is all that is necessary. After a colostomy, stoma care is needed.

3. While assessing a neonate with Hirschsprung's disease, it is important to keep in mind that 3.___
   I. symptoms usually begin at birth with a failure to pass meconium during the first 48 hours of life, often accompanied by abdominal distention and vomiting
   II. in the most severe cases, ischemic enterocolitis occurs and is manifested by acute abdominal distention, profuse vomiting, the passage of foul smelling gas, and large, loose, often bloody stools
   III. the infant deteriorates rapidly with a potentially lethal outcome if a colostomy is not performed immediately
   IV. in milder cases, chronic obstipation is the only symptom

The CORRECT answer is:
A. I, III B. I, II, III
C. II, III, IV D. II, IV

4. All of the following are appropriate surgical interventions for the treatment of Hirschsprung's disease in the newborn EXCEPT: 4.____
   A. A definitive pull-through procedure is delayed until 2 to 3 months of age, allowing the infant to reach an optimal nutritional state and the dilated bowel to return to normal size
   B. It is prudent to biopsy the colostomy to ensure that it does contain ganglion cells, as it will not function if aganglionosis exists at that site
   C. In the presence of ischemic enterocolitis, emergency colostomy is indicated
   D. Prior to the surgery, in infants with colitis, immediate resuscitation consists of passage of an orogastric tube, rapid vascular expansion, administration of antibiotics, and correction of acid-base deficits

5. The assessment findings in the neonate with meconium ileus include all of the following EXCEPT: 5.____
   A. Symptoms present as ileal obstruction 72 to 96 hours after birth and include increased abdominal girth, bilious vomiting, and the absence of stooling
   B. The anus and rectum are small in caliber and contain a small amount of gray meconium
   C. If the abdomen is not severely distended, the meconium may be palpated in dilated bowel loops as a doughy, rubbery mass on the right side of the abdomen
   D. Symptoms include abdominal distention within 24 hours of birth, respiratory distress, and prominent veins on an edematous, erythematous abdomen

6. Which of the following is NOT an appropriate surgical intervention for the treatment of meconium ileus in the newborn? 6.____
   A. The hyperosmolarity of administered gastrografin enema causes increased water return to the bowel lumen, which softens the meconium and facilitates passage.
   B. Resection of the obstructed segment, exteriorization of the affected segment, and postoperative irrigation are often required.
   C. Postoperatively, a nasogastric tube is connected to intermittent suction, and fluid maintenance offsets the fluid lost in the bowel.
   D. A sweat test, diagnostic for cystic fibrosis, is performed immediately after enterotomies.

7. Assessment findings in the neonate with pyloric stenosis include all of the following EXCEPT: 7.___
   A. It occurs four times more frequently in males than in females and is most often seen in the first born
   B. Vomiting usually begins at 6 weeks of age, increasing in frequency and force until there is projectile vomiting
   C. In 70% to 90% of patients, a small, firm, olive-size mass can often be palpated under the liver
   D. Gastric peristalsis may be seen as a wave progressing from the left upper quadrant to the right. Jaundice is associated in approximately 2% of these infants.

8. It is TRUE regarding appropriate surgical measures for the treatment of pyloric stenosis in the neonate that: 8.___
   I. The preoperative goal is to restore fluid and electrolyte balance. D_5 half normal saline infused at a rate of 100 ml/kg/8 hour with KCl added to equal 40 mEq/L usually restores balance within 12 to 48 hours
   II. The Rammstedt pyloromyotomy is done through a right transverse incision
   III. The hypertrophic muscle is split longitudinally, leaving the mucosa and submucosa intact
   IV. IV fluids are continued for 24 to 48 hours postoperatively, and oral feeds are resumed

   The CORRECT answer is:
   A. I, II, III
   B. I, III, IV
   C. II, IV
   D. I, II, III, IV

9. The assessment findings in the neonate with gastroesophageal reflux include all of the following EXCEPT: 9.___
   A. Vomiting is the most obvious sign of reflux and may prohibit adequate nutritional intake
   B. The gastric contents may be aspirated, causing frequent recurrent tumors
   C. Apnea and bradycardia, a more severe manifestation of aspiration, are triggered by even small amounts of gastric juices in or around the larynx
   D. Acidic fluid reflux into the esophagus may cause esophagitis, leading to anemia from bleeding, or may cause esophageal stricture formation

10. Which of the following is NOT an appropriate surgical intervention for the treatment of gastroesophageal reflux in the neonate? 10.___
   A. Preoperatively, renitidine or cimetidine will decrease the volume and acidity of gastric juice. Metoclopramide increases gastric emptying and improves lower esophageal sphincter function.
   B. Two weeks after the initial gastrostomy is done, a button gastrostomy can be placed.

C. Operations used in the treatment of reflux disease are the Nissen, Thal, and Boix-Ochoa fundoplication procedures. The common goal is to wrap the gastric fundus partially or completely around the gastro-esophageal junction to prevent reflux.
D. After an antireflux procedure, gastric decompression is continued for 1 to 2 days; then the gastrostomy tube is elevated for a day to ensure that the infant tolerates his or her own secretions.

11. Assessment findings in the neonate with biliary atresia include all of the following EXCEPT: 11.___
A. Biliary atresia is a dynamic disease process in which the disease progressively obliterates the bile ducts, with complete obliteration occurring at 9 to 12 months of age
B. Few newborns are visibly jaundiced
C. These infants often eat and grow normally until about 1 month of age, when scleral icterus and clay-colored stools may first be noticed
D. Hepatomegaly and splenomegaly

12. Which of the following is NOT an appropriate surgical intervention for the treatment of biliary atresia in the neonate? 12.___
A. If the intraoperative cholangiogram shows patency of the gallbladder, cystic duct, and distal common duct, the gallbladder can be anastomosed to the transected proximal hepatic duct at the liver hilus.
B. Usually, the gallbladder is small and fibrotic and a Kasai operation or hepatic portoenterostomy is indicated.
C. Kasai operation provides adequate bile drainage in approximately 90% of infants under 4 months of age.
D. Early diagnosis and operative intervention are essential because the success rate is inversely proportional to the infant's age.

13. The assessment findings in the neonate with necrotizing enterocolitis include 13.___
A. the product of a complicated pregnancy and/or a premature birth
B. apnea, bradycardia, and jaundice
C. bloody stools and localized abdominal erythema with induration
D. all of the above

14. All of the following are appropriate surgical interventions for the treatment of necrotizing enterocolitis in the neonate EXCEPT: 14.___
A. Preoperatively, parenteral antibiotics covering gram positive and gram negative organisms should be instituted. Pneumoperitoneum is an obvious indication for operative intervention.

B. At operation, frankly necrotic bowel requires resection with stoma formation or a primary anastomosis
C. Every effort should be made to preserve tracheoesophageal length
D. General supportive care with antibiotics, parenteral nutrition, and cardiorespiratory support is the mainstay of postoperative treatment

15. All of the following are high-risk factors for the neonate needing social work intervention EXCEPT 15.___
A. teenage pregnancy, ages 11 to 18
B. single parent; drug or alcohol abuse
C. mother or father with a history of being abused or early deprivation by own family, or history of having abused or neglected own children
D. attachment difficulties with neighbors

16. Which of the following is NOT a neonatal high-risk factor needing social work intervention? 16.___
A. Battered men
B. No prenatal care with previous or current pregnancies
C. Long-term hospitalization during pregnancy requiring intervention in helping family adjust
D. Other children with physical or mental handicaps

17. Which of the following pathologic grief factors related to perinatal loss are indications for referral for specialized care? 17.___
I. Acquisition of symptoms belonging to the last illness of the deceased
II. Formal manner resembling schizophrenia
III. Overactivity with a sense of loss
IV. Psychosomatic conditions such as ulcerative colitis and asthma

The CORRECT answer is:
A. I, II, III
B. I, II, IV
C. III, IV
D. I, II, III, IV

18. Since the child's understanding of death differs from that of adults, knowledge of the stages of growing awareness is essential for both parents and professionals working with children experiencing grief. 18.___
All of the following statements are correct concerning these stages EXCEPT:
A. In a toddler, age 1 to 3 years, no understanding of cause and effect of death is present
B. Preschoolers, age 3 to 6 years, view death as a temporary state and not an inevitable occurrence. They believe that they are the center of the universe and can do anything, and that thinking is doing.
C. School-age children, 6 to 12 years, understand that death is inevitable and irreversible
D. Adolescents, age over 12 years, are able to think abstractly about death like the adult

19. Of the following, the statement that provides INCORRECT information regarding pathologic grief as a result of perinatal loss is: 19.___
  A. Many people in grief-producing situations attempt to avoid the pain of grief and the expression of emotions which ultimately results in pathologic grief
  B. In many cases, the emotions accompanying unresolved grief may never be expressed and be forgotten by the unconscious mind
  C. Grief that is inhibited and never resolved is called abortive
  D. Chronic grief is characterized by an indefinite prolonging of the acute stage of depression. Chronic depression may be traceable to unresolved grief from the past.

20. Kinesthesis is the most natural pathway for fetal and neonatal growth and development. The interaction between infants and the extrauterine environment is also kinesthetic. 20.___
Tactile contact and vestibular stimulation are essential for all of the following EXCEPT
  A. organization and sorting of stimuli; coordination of sensory-motor skills
  B. a psychologic and social sense of self
  C. normal neurophysiologic development; normal body fluid electrolyte and acid-base balance
  D. emotional stability and temperament

21. It is NOT true regarding appropriate measures for care-giving in different newborn states that in 21.___
  A. deep sleep state term babies may exhibit a *slow* heart rate of 100 to 110 beats/minute which should trigger heart rate alarms and result in necessary stimulation by NICU staff
  B. light sleep state babies may cry or fuss and be awakened to feed before they are truly awake and ready to eat
  C. quiet alert state baby is maximally able to attend and reciprocally respond to parents. This is the best state for interaction with parents.
  D. crying state, talking, holding, rocking, or putting baby upright on caretaker's shoulder may quiet infant

22. Circadian rhythms are cyclic variations in function that occur daily 22.___
  A. between 12 A.M. and 8 A.M.
  B. between 8 A.M. and 4 P.M.
  C. between 4 P.M. and 12 P.M.
  D. at about the same time

23. All of the following are correct about tactile and kinesthesis in the newborn EXCEPT: 23.___
   A. Touch is the major method of communication for neonates and infants
   B. The senses of touch, temperature, and pressure are all well developed and receptors lie in the newborn's skin
   C. The sensitivity to touch is especially well-developed in the face, around the lips, and in the hands
   D. Babies are not barometers for adult feelings. The baby does not know if the adult is tired and irritable and does not respond with irritability or crying

24. A noise level *too loud* for both the preonates and the neonates is prohibited since the human cochlea has normal adult function and is sensitive to noise after _____ weeks' gestation. 24.___
   A. 20 B. 24 C. 28 D. 32

25. The developmental stage that has been described in the communication process between preonates and their mothers is known as the _____ stage. 25.___
   A. physiologic B. behavioral
   C. sympathetic D. all of the above

KEY (CORRECT ANSWERS)

1. D
2. C
3. B
4. A
5. A

6. D
7. B
8. A
9. B
10. B

11. A
12. C
13. D
14. C
15. D

16. A
17. B
18. A
19. B
20. C

21. A
22. D
23. D
24. A
25. D

TEST 2

DIRECTIONS: Each question or incomplete statement is followed by several suggested answers or completions. Select the one that BEST answers the question or completes the statement. *PRINT THE LETTER OF THE CORRECT ANSWER IN THE SPACE AT THE RIGHT.*

1. Which of the following is NOT true about one of the caretaker factors? 1.___
   A. Parental expectations have a major effect on their perceptions and behavior, and ultimately affect the child's development.
   B. If the pregnancy has failed to produce a normal, healthy baby, the parents must grieve the loss of their expectations. Parents are unable to attach to and take care of the baby until they have completed their grief work.
   C. Consistency in maternal responses is especially important as the infant continues to learn the accepted patterns of cues from the caretaker.
   D. Multiple caretaking improves establishment of bio-rhythms for sleep-awake cycles, feeding, and visual attentiveness.

2. All of the following are appropriate interventions for babies in the NICU EXCEPT: 2.___
   A. The first goal in auditory intervention is to assess the current level of noise in the NICU and to decrease the noise decibels wherever possible
   B. The first goal in visual intervention is to assess the current level of light and increase it wherever possible
   C. Enhancing the olfactory environment includes having parents hold the infant or sit close if the infant cannot yet be held
   D. Immediate response to crying decreases the infant's physiologic stress, increases the infant's trust in the environment, and enhances the sense of self and of control over the world

3. Which of the following is an INAPPROPRIATE auditory intervention in the NICU? 3.___
   A. The NICU is a noisy environment that has no diurnal rhythm. The NICU infant is exposed to an onslaught of noise 24 hours a day.
   B. No tapping or banging on the incubator plexiglas should ever be permitted.
   C. If music is played in the NICU, it should be below 50-60 dB, should not be rock music, and preferably should be classical.
   D. All newborns, except those with hyperbilirubinemia, congenital viral infections, and those receiving atotoxic drugs, should have a hearing screening before discharge.

4. Which of the following is an APPROPRIATE strategy to facilitate nipple feeding in high-risk neonates? 4.____
   A. Suction only routinely, consider indwelling gastric tube rather than intermittent gavage, use only orthodontic nipples/pacifiers if mother wants to breastfeed.
   B. Have baby smell/taste breast milk, facilitate hand-to-mouth behaviors, use Lact-Aid nursing supplementer.
   C. Semireclining on lap of caretaker, gentle tugging at nipple causes baby to stop sucking.
   D. All of the above

5. All of the following are correct about the steps followed in *Tommy's feeding plan* to facilitate nipple feeding EXCEPT: 5.____
   A. Sit upright, which decreases the flow of formula from the bottle, and thus decreases gag reflex which causes bradycardia and anxiety
   B. Use a brown nipple, which is the shortest nipple and decreases stimulation of hypersensitive gag reflex
   C. Gently push up under his chin when he gets a mouthful of formula
   D. Talk to him softly and gently telling him that he can swallow and praise him when he does

6. Which of the following define *ethics* in neonatal intensive care APPROPRIATELY? 6.____
   I. Ethics is the study of rational processes for determining the most morally desirable course of action in view of conflicting value choices.
   II. Ethics is a branch of psychosociology that considers competing values in order to obtain the best possible outcome to a given situation.
   III. The most morally desirable course of action is determined by whether, and how, that action adheres to the ethical principles held by those involved in making decisions.
   IV. When values conflict and each value is morally justifiable, an ethical dilemma exists. For an ethical dilemma to exist, a real choice between possible courses of action must exist.

   The CORRECT answer is:
   A. I, II, III B. II, III, IV
   C. I, III, IV D. I, II, III, IV

7. Which of the following is NOT true of nursing ethics in neonatal intensive care? 7.____
   A. It is not always the nurse's obligation to make sure the patient's best interests are being met since the nurse simply has to follow whatever instructions are given by the physician.
   B. If the physician makes an unsound medical judgment, it is the nurse's obligation to clarify the intention and correct the situation if necessary.

C. Moral dilemma can face nurses when their moral values conflict with the physician's or the parents' or when their professional obligations conflict with those of their chosen moral community. Important decisions must be made by nurses during conflicts of this sort.

D. No one in the health care team is required to ignore his or her personal values if deep conflict exists. A nurse, as well as any other health care professional, may withdraw from a case.

8. Once fetal asphyxia is diagnosed, therapeutic interventions should be coordinated to allow for a timely delivery and effective, coordinated resuscitation. The BASIC goal of resuscitation is to 8.___

A. maintain adequate cardiac output and tissue perfusion
B. maintain normal core temperature and avoid hypoglycemia while stabilizing the infant for transport to the nursery
C. expand the lungs and maintain adequate ventilation and oxygenation
D. all of the above

9. Of the following, the ABSOLUTE indicator of the neonate being in shock in the delivery room is 9.___

A. bradycardia
B. hypotension
C. poor peripheral perfusion, pallor, and decreased capillary filling
D. none of the above

10. External cardiac compression to the neonate in shock is REQUIRED when the heart rate is less than or equal to _____ beats/minute or less than _____ beats/minute with at least 30 seconds of supported effective ventilation provided. 10.___

A. 70; 90 B. 60; 80 C. 50; 70 D. 40; 60

11. Which of the following is NOT an appropriate laboratory data that should be used to evaluate neonatal metabolic derangements associated with thermal instability? 11.___

A. Complete blood count to assess for sepsis
B. Blood galactose level to assess for hypoglycemia
C. Arterial blood gas to assess for hypoxemia and metabolic acidosis
D. Serum and urine osmolality to assess hydration and electrolytes to assess for hyperkalemia

12. An exchange transfusion should be performed immediately to severely anemic neonates with a hemoglobin concentration of less than 12 g/dl, edema or hepatosplenomegaly. This transfusion should be a 12.___

A. partial exchange transfusion with 30 ml/kg of red cells followed by a full exchange transfusion when the neonate is stable

B. transfusion with 40 ml/kg of packed red cells
C. partial exchange transfusion with 40 ml/kg of packed red cells followed by a full exchange transfusion when the neonate is stable
D. transfusion with 30 ml/kg of packed red cells

13. Severe _____ is suggested by a positive direct Coombs' test in ABO hemolytic disease. 13.___
A. hyperbilirubinemia
B. reticulocytosis and spherocytosis
C. RH incompatibility
D. hemolysis

14. Giving RhoGAM to an RH-negative mother within _____ day(s) of delivery of an RH-positive infant or fetus, if an abortion, prevents MOST cases of erythroblastosis fetalis. 14.___
A. one B. two C. three D. four

15. If acute blood loss is suspected and the neonate is pale and limp at birth, blood pressure should be obtained and monitored, oxygen should be administered, and intravenous fluids should be started at _____ ml/kg. 15.___
A. 20 B. 30 C. 40 D. 50

16. During the neonatal blood transfusion, the nurse should be familiar with the information that it is NOT appropriate for the blood to hang for more than _____ hours. 16.___
A. 1 to 3 B. 3 to 5 C. 4 to 6 D. 6 to 8

17. The MOST appropriate needle size to administer fresh blood to the neonate without significant hemolysis is _____-gauge. 17.___
A. 20 B. 25 C. 30 D. 35

18. The newborn with a bleeding problem who looks well and does not appear ill suggests all of the following causes of bleeding EXCEPT 18.___
A. vitamin K deficiency
B. platelet defect
C. sepsis
D. hemophilia or other hereditary factor deficiency

19. The IDEAL product for treating hemophilia A in infants once it is licensed which also avoids all risk of viral infection is _____ concentrate. 19.___
A. factor III B. recombinant factor XIII
C. factor IX D. recombinant factor VIII

20. How many units of factor VIII equal one pack of cryoprecipitate? 20.___
A. 100 B. 200 C. 300 D. 400

21. Isoimmune thrombocytopenia has an 80% chance of recurrence in subsequent pregnancies. 21.___
A fetal platelet count ABOVE _____/mm^3 would suggest a safe vaginal delivery.
A. 20,000 B. 30,000 C. 60,000 D. 80,000

22. Visible icterus appears first on the head and face. 22.___
Of the following body parts, the LAST skin surface to be affected is the
A. abdomen B. back C. chest D. extremities

23. Heparinized blood must be used within _____ hours of preparation of the unit in exchange transfusion of jaundiced infants. 23.___
A. 12 B. 24 C. 48 D. 72

24. The PRIMARY serologic laboratory test used to identify HIV in the neonate is 24.___
A. HIV-specific IgA test
B. polymerase chain reaction test
C. P24 antigen test
D. enzyme-linked immunosorbent assay

25. Assessment findings in the neonate with rubella virus include all of the following EXCEPT 25.___
A. intracerebral calcification
B. cataracts and purpura
C. microcephaly and cardiac defects
D. hepatosplenomegaly

KEY (CORRECT ANSWERS)

1. D
2. B
3. D
4. B
5. B

6. C
7. A
8. D
9. D
10. B

11. B
12. C
13. D
14. C
15. A

16. C
17. B
18. C
19. D
20. A

21. B
22. D
23. B
24. D
25. A

EXAMINATION SECTION
TEST 1

DIRECTIONS: Each question or incomplete statement is followed by several suggested answers or completions. Select the one that BEST answers the question or completes the statement. *PRINT THE LETTER OF THE CORRECT ANSWER IN THE SPACE AT THE RIGHT.*

1. Which of the following is NOT an appropriate pathophysiologic finding for neurogenic bladder in the neonate? 1.____
   A. Neurogenic bladder is an anatomic interruption of the micturition reflex normally triggered by a full bladder.
   B. Upper motor neuron deficit causes bladder atony and lower motor neuron deficit can cause spasticity.
   C. Diagnosis begins immediately at the bedside when the newborn has no apparent voiding stream or the urine flow rate falls below expectations without other explanations.
   D. Diagnosis is further clarified by voiding cystourethrogram and by cystometric studies.

2. All of the following are appropriate measures in the treatment of neurogenic bladder in the neonate EXCEPT: 2.____
   A. If a VCUG shows no reflux and the urine appears to flow freely from the bladder with only a small amount of residual urine, no intervention is necessary
   B. If the sphincter tone is such that urine is stagnant in the bladder, gentle Crede's maneuver at regular intervals can be initiated. Crede's maneuver should be performed only after a VCUG has documented a severe reflux.
   C. Surgical intervention is indicated when there is severe reflux with renal damage present or recurrent UTI.
   D. The urologist creates a vesicostomy to allow the free flow of urine into diapers

3. Holoprosencephaly, one of the serious neurologic segmentation defects, is characterized by 3.____
   A. a single, midline, lateral ventricle
   B. complete interhemispheric fissure
   C. midfacial clefts and hypertolerism
   D. all of the above

4. Neurologic migrational anomalies in the neonate easily lead to problems of gray matter dysfunction. Common manifestations in the newborn period include all of the following EXCEPT 4.____
   A. seizures and abnormal cry
   B. meningocephaly
   C. small-for-gestational age (SGA)
   D. abnormal transillumination

5. Clinical features of porencephaly in the neonate include all of the following EXCEPT 5.____
   A. seizures
   B. motor problems
   C. abnormal transillumination if the cyst is superficial
   D. decreased intracranial pressure if the cyst is enlarging

6. Clinical features of lissencephaly in the neonate do NOT include 6.____
   A. seizures and large-for-gestational age (LGA)
   B. microcephaly and polyhydramnios
   C. micrognathia and downward-slanted palpebral fissures
   D. anteverted nares and prominent forehead and occiput

7. Clinical features of neonatal macrogyria in the newborn period include 7.____
   A. spastic hemiplegia
   B. spastic diplegia
   C. mental retardation
   D. none of the above

8. Signs and symptoms of absence of the corpus callosum in the newborn are most often a result of associated malformations and anomalies. 8.____
   These include all of the following EXCEPT
   A. seizures and mental retardation
   B. hydrocephalus
   C. sensory dysfunctions
   D. asynchronous electroencephalogram

9. Clinical features of the Dandy-Walker cyst, a cerebellar malformation in the neonate do NOT include 9.____
   A. frequent progressive hydrocephalus and enlargement of the occipital shelf and posterior part of the skull
   B. positive transillumination in a triangular shape
   C. nystagmus and lateral gaze palsy
   D. respiratory control abnormalities and micrognathia

10. Craniosynostosis in the neonate should be suspected in the presence of microcephaly or a misshapen head. 10.____
    Appropriate evaluation requires
    I. x-ray films of the skull
    II. CT scan
    III. electrocraniosynostogram

    The CORRECT answer is:
    A. I, II
    B. I, III
    C. II *only*
    D. II, III

11. Which of the following tests have become MOST helpful in recent years allowing for prenatal diagnosis of certain congenital malformations of the nervous system? 11.____
    A. X-ray films and CT scan
    B. CT scan and ultrasound examination

C. Ultrasound examination and determination of alpha-fetoprotein in the amniotic fluid
D. All of the above

12. Very limited treatment is available for congenital malformations of the nervous system. 12.___
All of the following are appropriate strategies for making efforts at reducing secondary complications or providing earlier management to handle these complications more efficiently EXCEPT:
A. When treatment is thought to be appropriate, closure of the myelomeningocele should be performed as soon as possible to reduce the risk of meningitis and ventriculitis. Shunting becomes necessary if the infant develops hydrocephalus after the closure of the primary defect.
B. The only situation in which microcephaly is considered treatable is total craniosynostosis
C. The management of congenital hydrocephalus consists primarily of early shunting, between 7 and 14 days of age
D. If the encephalocele is small and a large amount of the brain is not contained in the sac, the defect should be closed

13. All of the following are symptoms of increased intracranial pressure to be observed and assessed after a ventriculoperitoneal shunt EXCEPT 13.___
A. increasing head circumference
B. poor feeding
C. sunset sign of eyes
D. pallor

14. Of the following, only _____ is NOT among the most commonly encountered forms of extracranial hemorrhage that are distinguished not only in clinical manifestations but also in pathophysiology. 14.___
A. intraspinal hemorrhage
B. caput succedaneum
C. subgaleal hemorrhage
D. cephalhematoma

15. The typical depressed skull fracture in the newborn is of the *ping-pong* type, an indentation without loss of bony continuity. 15.___
When neurologic signs are present, _____ should be suspected.
A. direct cerebral injury
B. intracranial bleeding
C. free bone fragments
D. all of the above

16. Occipital osteodiastasis is a traumatic separation of the squamous and lateral portions of the occipital bone. 16.___
It is identified ONLY by
A. x-ray films
B. autopsy
C. ultrasound
D. CT scan

17. The MOST common type of neonatal intracranial hemorrhage is 17.___
    A. subarachnoid hemorrhage
    B. subdural hemorrhage
    C. intracerebellar hematoma
    D. epidural hematoma

18. Surgical evacuation of _____ clots may be necessary as an emergency procedure in the neonatal intracranial hemorrhage. 18.___
    A. cerebral   B. cerebellar
    C. epidural and subdural   D. subgaleal and occipital

19. Clinical manifestations of neonatal spinal cord injuries depend on the severity and location of the injury. Clinical syndromes include all of the following EXCEPT 19.___
    A. stillbirth or rapid neonatal death
    B. spinal shock syndrome
    C. Horner's syndrome
    D. respiratory failure

20. Clinical syndromes of neonatal plexus injuries do NOT include 20.___
    A. Erb's palsy, which accounts for about 90% of plexus injuries
    B. total palsy, which occurs in 8% to 9% of cases
    C. Klumpke's paralysis, which is seen in less than 2% of cases
    D. none of the above

21. Treatment of the neonatal plexus injuries should include immobilization for _____ days. 21.___
    A. 1 to 2   B. 3 to 4   C. 5 to 6   D. 7 to 10

22. All of the following statements are true regarding the common causes of neonatal seizures EXCEPT: 22.___
    A. Acute metabolic conditions include hypocalcemia, hypomagnesemia, hyponatremia, and pyridoxine dependency or deficiency
    B. Intracranial hemorrhage includes subdural hematoma, subarachnoid hemorrhage, epidural hemorrhage, and subgaleal hemorrhage
    C. Infections include viral encephalitis, bacterial meningitis, sepsis, and brain abscess
    D. Inherited metabolic conditions include maple syrup urine disease, nonketotic hyperglycemia, galactosemia, and organic acidemias

23. The CLASSICAL categories of neonatal seizures are 23.___
    I. clonic   II. subtonic
    III. tonic   IV. myoclonic

    The CORRECT answer is:
    A. I, II   B. I, II, III
    C. I, III, IV   D. II, IV

24. Which of the following is NOT an appropriate measure for the acute management of neonatal seizures? 24.____
   A. Draw blood for glucose, calcium, magnesium, blood gas analysis, and electrolytes.
   B. Maintain adequate oxygenation and ventilation.
   C. If dextrostix is less than 25-45, give 200 mg/kg IV minibolus of glucose.
   D. If dextrostix is more than 25-45, give phenobarbital 80 mg/kg IV.

25. Though no ideal classification has yet been possible, a classification based on the extent of hemorrhage seen on the CT scan grades germinal matrix hemorrhages in all of the following categories EXCEPT 25.____
   A. I: No bleeding
   B. II: Germinal matrix with blood in the ventricles
   C. III: Germinal matrix with blood in the ventricles and hydrocephalus
   D. IV: Intraventricular and parenchymal bleeding, other than germinal matrix

KEY (CORRECT ANSWERS)

1. B
2. B
3. A
4. B
5. D

6. A
7. D
8. C
9. D
10. A

11. C
12. C
13. D
14. A
15. D

16. B
17. A
18. C
19. C
20. D

21. D
22. B
23. C
24. D
25. A

TEST 2

DIRECTIONS: Each question or incomplete statement is followed by several suggested answers or completions. Select the one that BEST answers the question or completes the statement. *PRINT THE LETTER OF THE CORRECT ANSWER IN THE SPACE AT THE RIGHT.*

1. Assessment findings in neonates with neurologic intraventricular hemorrhage include all of the following EXCEPT: 1.____
   A. Some infants, generally those who are at term, will have intraventricular hemorrhages associated with severe asphyxia
   B. Premature infants often show shock, respiratory distress syndrome, coagulopathy, hyperviscosity, hypoxia, gestational age more than 40 weeks, and birth asphyxia
   C. Common signs of germinal matrix hemorrhage include apnea, hypotension, drop in hematocrit, flaccidity, areflexia, full fontanel, tonic posturing
   D. In the case of periventricular-intraventricular hemorrhage, both ultrasonography and CT scanning are useful tools for defining the presence of bleeding and for following its evolution

2. The TRUE statements regarding appropriate treatment and intervention measures for the management of neonatal neurologic intraventricular hemorrhage are: 2.____
   I. The removal of blood from the ventricular system has been used for many years as a treatment for intraventricular hemorrhage
   II. Care must be given to reduce the risk for continued bleeding, working to maintain perfusion of the brain and to reduce wide fluctuations in blood pressure, oxygenation, and pH
   III. Lumbar puncture has much less chance of morbidity and is the preferred procedure. Ventricular taps are also among the recommended ones.
   IV. Medications to reduce intracranial pressure and therefore treat secondary effects of the bleeding include furosemide, acetazolamide, and steroid agents

   The CORRECT answer is:
   A. I, II, III　　B. I, II, IV
   C. I, III, IV　　D. II, III, IV

3. Common risk factors for abnormal neurologic development include all of the following EXCEPT 3.____
   A. hyperglycemia and polycythemia
   B. seizures and inappropriate size for gestational age
   C. asphyxia and prematurity
   D. birth trauma and maternal drug abuse

4. Chromosomal aberrations should be suspected in all of the following situations EXCEPT 4.____
   A. large-for-gestational-age weight, length, and/or head circumference
   B. presence of dysmorphic features
   C. neurologic and/or neuromuscular dysfunction
   D. family history of multiple miscarriages or siblings with mental retardation or birth defects

5. As a rule, numeric chromosomal abnormalities are NOT associated with 5.____
   A. intrauterine growth retardation
   B. dysmorphic features and malformations
   C. ornithine transcarbamylase deficiency (OTC)
   D. mental retardation

6. All of the following are true about Down's syndrome EXCEPT: 6.____
   A. It has an incidence of approximately 1 in 600 live births
   B. The classic phenotype includes simian creases, single flexion creases, and incurving of the fifth fingers, and increased distance between the 1st and 2nd toes
   C. The classic phenotype includes a flattened occiput, midfacial hypoplasia, depressed nasal bridge, epicanthic folds, micrognathia, and excess nuchal skin
   D. Approximately 95% of cases are caused by nondisjunction involving chromosome 21; 5% are caused by a mosaicism; and 1% have a translocation

7. Which of the following is NOT true about Turner syndrome? 7.____
   A. The only monosomy to be seen in live births is that of Turner syndrome - females with a 45,X karyotype.
   B. It is the only numeric abnormality of the sex chromosome that may be identifiable at birth. Turner syndrome has an incidence of 1 in 1000 female births.
   C. Clinical features in the newborn period are a short, webbed neck, and marked lymphedema of the dorsum of the hands and feet.
   D. Congenital heart defects are seen in about half the patients. Intelligence is normal and prognosis is usually excellent.

8. Regarding Cri du chat syndrome, it is TRUE that: 8.____
   I. These infants are usually large for gestational age, hypertonic, and microcephalic
   II. This syndrome is the result of loss of the terminal end of the short arm of chromosome 5. These infants have an unusual cat-like weak cry in the neonatal period
   III. The classic phenotype includes epicanthic folds, ocular hypertolerism, low-set ears, and micrognathia
   IV. Mental retardation is rarely seen

   The CORRECT answer is:
   A. I, II
   B. I, III, IV
   C. II, III
   D. II, III, IV

9. All of the following are major characteristics of autosomal recessive inheritance EXCEPT 9.___
   A. phenotypically abnormal parents
   B. both males and females affected
   C. increased incidence of consanguinity
   D. offspring of two carrier parents are at a 25% risk of being affected. Unaffected siblings have a two-thirds chance of being carriers.

10. All of the following are true of X-linked recessive disorders EXCEPT: 10.___
   A. They are phenotypically expressed in hemizygous males. Heterozygous females are generally phenotypically normal and are referred to as carriers.
   B. Affected fathers do not have affected sons; however, all daughters of affected males are carriers.
   C. A carrier female has a 25% chance of having an affected male offspring
   D. X-linked recessive disorders that may be recognizable in the newborn period include factor VIII and IX deficiency, X-linked hydrocephalus, and Opitz syndrome

11. Which of the following is NOT correct about X-linked dominant disorders? 11.___
   A. They occur when the abnormal gene located on the X chromosome is expressed in both the hemizygous and heterozygous states.
   B. There is no male-to-male transmission but all daughters of an affected male will be affected.
   C. Disorders that are known to be inherited as X-linked dominant include incontinentia pigmenti, ornithine transcarbamylase deficiency (OTC), and hypophosphatemia.
   D. Early diagnosis of OTC is important because, if untreated, it leads to neonatal hyperammonemia and death in affected females.

12. Recurrence risks in multifactorial genetic disorders are not constant as in single-gene disorders, but are influenced by 12.___
   I. the number of family members affected
   II. the degree of relatedness to those affected
   III. the cause of the defect
   IV. the sex of the individual

   The CORRECT answer is:
   A. I, II, III B. I, III
   C. I, II, IV D. II, III, IV

13. Laboratory studies that should be obtained before any treatment is begun in the neonate are electrolytes, ammonia, glucose, urine pH, urine-reducing substances, and urine ketones. 13.___

Clues to suspecting an inborn error include
A. hypoglycemia and ketonuria
B. acidosis with recurrent vomiting and hyperammonemia
C. acidosis that is difficult to correct and is out of proportion to the clinical state
D. all of the above

14. Environmental exposures may have adverse effects on fetal development, resulting in malformations and neurodevelopmental abnormalities in infants and children. Of the following, only _____ is(are) NOT teratogenic in humans. 14.___
A. alcohol and cocaine
B. anticonvulsants
C. adenosine deaminase
D. isotretinoin

15. Human teratogenic agents are divided into all of the following categories EXCEPT 15.___
A. bacterial agents
B. chemical agents
C. radiation
D. maternal factors

16. Of the following, the INAPPROPRIATE laboratory finding in the bowel problem of the newborn known as malrotation and volvulus is: 16.___
A. Plain films of the abdomen show a dilated duodenum and proximal stomach
B. An upper GI series will confirm the point of partial obstruction and an abnormal ligament of Treitz. A barium enema will also show an abnormal rotation.
C. In midgut volvulus, plain abdominal films show gastric and duodenal distention. These infants should have an emergency barium enema that will show the colon's occlusion at the point it twists around the mesenteric vessels.
D. Severe acid-base derangement may be seen if there is significant bowel necrosis

17. Which of the following is NOT an appropriate treatment measure for the management of malrotation and volvulus in the newborn? 17.___
A. Correction of electrolyte and acid-base abnormalities and parenteral antibiotics instituted in the preoperative period
B. Gastric decompression and vigorous fluid hydration in the postoperative period
C. Emergency abdominal exploration for the infant with volvulus because the bowel will be irreparably damaged within 4 hours
D. Operative correction for malrotation including division of Ladd's bands to relieve the duodenal obstruction and placement of the colon in the left side of the abdomen and the small bowel on the right

18. All of the following are signs and symptoms of omphalocele and gastroschisis in the newborn EXCEPT: 18.___
   A. Both of these are defects in the abdominal wall around the umbilicus. Both present as a mass of abdominal contents extruding through an anterior abdominal wall defect.
   B. Gastroschisis patients have only bowel eviscerated
   C. Omphaloceles, including bowel evisceration, may also contain liver
   D. Gastroschisis is always to the left of the midline and will often have a skin bridge between the umbilicus and the defect

19. Of the following surgical interventions for the treatment of omphalocele and gastroschisis in the newborn, the INAPPROPRIATE one is: 19.___
   A. Preoperative care includes preservation of body heat, gastric decompression, protection of the intestine, and prophylaxis against infection
   B. Heat and fluid loss are minimized by wrapping the herniated abdominal contents with warm, saline-soaked gauze and plastic wrap
   C. Omphalocele patients are never too ill to undergo operation or have other malformations inconsistent with long-term survival
   D. Primary surgical repair entails placing the abdominal contents into the abdominal cavity without increasing abdominal pressure to the point that ventilation, venous return, or intestinal blood supply is compromised

20. All of the following are expected signs and symptoms of diaphragmatic hernia in the newborn EXCEPT 20.___
   A. respiratory distress immediately after birth
   B. scaphoid abdomen and an increased anteroposterior diameter of the chest
   C. associated anomalies including hypoplasia of the lung, malrotation of the intestine, and patent ductus arteriosus
   D. loud breath sounds on the affected side and the mediastinum placed toward the contralateral side

21. APPROPRIATE surgical measurements for the management of diaphragmatic hernia in the newborn include: 21.___
   I. The principal postoperative concern is hemorrhage
   II. As soon as the disorder is suspected, an orogastric tube should be placed for gastric decompression
   III. The abdominal contents are reduced from the chest and replaced into the abdominal cavity, and the diaphragmatic defect is closed
   IV. An endotracheal tube is placed on the affected side

   The CORRECT answer is:
   A. I, II
   B. I, II, III
   C. II, III
   D. II, IV

22. The assessment findings in the neonate with esophageal atresia (EA) include all of the following EXCEPT: 22.____
   A. Most infants present soon after birth with copious secretions or inability to swallow feedings
   B. After one or two sucks, the child will begin coughing and then regurgitate unchanged formula. An orogastric tube should be passed and will meet an obstruction at 25 to 35 cm from the mouth if esophageal atresia is present.
   C. Patients with upper pouch fistulas will aspirate feedings
   D. Infants with an *H* type fistula may have a more insidious onset of symptoms. They will cough and choke with feeding and may have intermittent abdominal distention or recurrent pneumonia over the first months of life.

23. Which of the following is NOT an appropriate surgical intervention for the treatment of newborns with esophageal atresia and associated fistula? 23.____
   A. Once the diagnosis is established, the catheter in the upper pouch should be placed on suction to prevent aspiration. An urgent operation is indicated if a proximal fistula is present.
   B. The surgical repair of standard esophageal atresia should be carried out as soon as the patient is stable.
   C. After a wait of several days to as long as 16 weeks to allow maximal growth of the distal esophagus, a second operation completes the repair.
   D. Postoperative care includes pulmonary toilet, IV fluids, and antibiotics.

24. The assessment findings in the neonate with bowel atresia and stenosis include which of the following? 24.____
   I. Typically, the neonate is small for gestational age and the mother has polyhydramnios.
   II. The more distal the atresia the more likely the polyhydramnios.
   III. The infant has bilious vomiting and abdominal distention. If the atresia occurs late in gestation, the infant will not pass meconium.
   IV. Duodenal atresia is frequently associated with trisomy 21.

   The CORRECT answer is:
   A. I, II   B. I, IV
   C. II, III, IV   D. I, II, III, IV

25. All of the following are appropriate surgical interventions for the treatment of bowel atresia and stenosis in the neonate EXCEPT: 25.___

A. Jejunoileal atresias are repaired by a simple right retropleural anastomosis
B. Duodenal atresia often requires repair through a side-to-side anastomosis to prevent injury to the bile and pancreatic ducts
C. Preoperative care includes gastric decompression, intravenous hydration, and replacement of electrolytes
D. Postoperatively, the bowel is decompressed by an OG tube until bowel function begins

KEY (CORRECT ANSWERS)

1. B
2. B
3. A
4. A
5. C

6. D
7. B
8. C
9. A
10. C

11. D
12. C
13. D
14. C
15. A

16. A
17. B
18. D
19. C
20. D

21. C
22. B
23. C
24. B
25. A

EXAMINATION SECTION
TEST 1

DIRECTIONS: Each question or incomplete statement is followed by several suggested answers or completions. Select the one that BEST answers the question or completes the statement. *PRINT THE LETTER OF THE CORRECT ANSWER IN THE SPACE AT THE RIGHT.*

1. The assessment findings of Ebstein's anomaly include all of the following EXCEPT: 1.___
   A. In severely affected infants, the amount of pulmonary blood flow is markedly decreased and these infants may be deeply cyanotic
   B. The second heart sound, S_2, is normal in the mildly affected infant, but the pulmonary component of S_2 may be diminished or inaudible in severely affected patients
   C. Diastolic murmurs, ejection clicks, and triple or quadruple rhythms are rarely heard
   D. Symptomatic newborns usually have congestive heart failure resulting from volume overload of the left ventricle

2. In the infant with Ebstein's anomaly, 2.___
   A. the PaO_2 may be normal to very high, depending on the amount of blood flow through the pulmonary valve
   B. the chest x-ray shows cardiomegaly with decreased pulmonary vascularity
   C. an electrocardiogram shows abnormal P waves and various degrees of heart block, frequent presence of Wolff-Parkinson-White syndrome, dysrhythmias, and the QRS generally showing a right bundle-branch block pattern
   D. an echocardiogram with abnormal tricuspid valve patterns on an M mode suggests Ebstein's anomaly. A two-dimensional echocardiogram is diagnostic.

3. All of the following are true statements concerning infants with complete D-transposition of the great arteries EXCEPT: 3.___
   A. It is more prevalent in males and is typically found in infants who are full-term
   B. The major physiologic abnormalities are an oxygen deficiency in the tissues and excessive work load of the right and left ventricles
   C. The S_2 is single with an increased intensity. Murmurs, if present, are usually those of associated lesions.
   D. No signs of congestive heart failure are present. Digoxin should be used if subvalvular pulmonary stenosis is present.

4. Which of the following is NOT an appropriate laboratory finding in the infant with complete D-transposition of the great arteries? 4.____
   A. The pH and $PaCO_2$ are normal. The PaO_2 is typically low but if a large VSD or PDA is present, the PaO_2 may approach normal levels.
   B. In chest x-ray, the cardiac silhouette may assume the shape of an egg lying on a string, which is diagnostic.
   C. The electrocardiogram may be normal or show right ventricular hypertrophy.
   D. The echocardiogram is extremely useful in establishing the diagnosis and evaluating associated lesions.

5. In the surgical treatment of infants with complete D-transposition of the great arteries, the arterial switch procedure 5.____
   I. is the treatment of choice in most centers
   II. through a median sternotomy incision involves amputation of the main pulmonary artery and the aorta below the respective valves
   III. consists of the pulmonary artery being anastomosed to the left ventricle and the aorta anastomosed to the right ventricle
   IV. and the Mustard and Senning procedures are the most common

   The CORRECT answer is:
   A. I, II B. I, II, III
   C. I, IV D. III, IV

6. Tetralogy of Fallot is the most common form of cyanotic congenital heart disease. 6.____
   _____ is NOT one of the components of Tetralogy of Fallot.
   A. Ventricular septal defect
   B. Overriding of the descending aorta
   C. Obstruction to the right ventricular outflow tract
   D. Right ventricular hypertrophy

7. Assessment findings in neonates with Tetralogy of Fallot include all of the following EXCEPT 7.____
   A. severe right ventricular outflow tract obstruction
   B. the predominant intercardiac shunt is right to left; therefore, most infants are cyanotic
   C. the S_2 is usually loud and single, representing aortic closure
   D. congestive heart failure

8. Which of the following is NOT an appropriate laboratory finding in the infant with Tetralogy of Fallot? 8.____
   A. The $PaCO_2$ and pH are normal. If the pulmonary stenosis is very severe, the amount of right-to-left shunting increases and the PaO_2 increases too.

B. The classic chest x-ray resembles the shape of a boot with a normal-sized heart; however, this pattern is not common in the newborn.
C. The electrocardiogram demonstrates right ventricular hypertrophy.
D. Echocardiograms help identify the pulmonary valve to rule out pulmonary atresia. Doppler interrogation helps to define the degree and level of pulmonary stenosis.

9. The INCORRECT statement about the treatment of Tetralogy of Fallot in neonates is: 9.____
A. Propranolol is the preferable drug for treating hypercyanotic infants, although morphine has been used successfully
B. Total surgical repair involves patch closure of the large VSD and relief of the right ventricular outflow obstruction performed through a median sternotomy incision
C. Contraindications of surgical treatment include small size of the child, anomalous right anterior ascending coronary artery, and hypoplastic pulmonary arteries
D. Total surgical repair is not usually recommended in the neonatal period

10. Complications and residual effects of Tetralogy of Fallot include all of the following EXCEPT 10.____
A. diminished or absent pulses in the affected arm
B. congestive heart failure from an overlarge shunt
C. inadequate shunt
D. mortality in infancy of 40%

11. Pulmonary atresia with intact ventricular septum is characterized by COMPLETE agenesis of the pulmonary 11.____
A. artery
B. vein
C. valve
D. all of the above

12. Assessment findings in infants with pulmonary atresia include all of the following EXCEPT: 12.____
A. Cyanosis is always present in varying degrees, depending on the amount of pulmonary blood flow from the PDA
B. Cyanosis is always present in varying degrees, depending on the collateral blood flow
C. The S_2 is single, and a soft systolic murmur is heard as a result of either the PDA or mitral insufficiency in about one-third of infants with pulmonary atresia
D. Congestive heart failure is usually present with moderate to severe tricuspid insufficiency

13. Which of the following is NOT an appropriate laboratory finding in the infant with pulmonary atresia? 13.___
   A. The pH and $PaCO_2$ are usually above normal range, the PaO_2 is usually very low, unless there is a large shunt at the ductal or bronchial collateral level.
   B. In chest x-ray, the heart appears enlarged if tricuspid insufficiency is present. Pulmonary vascularity is either increased or normal.
   C. The electrocardiogram is usually abnormal, but may show left ventricular hypertrophy.
   D. The two-dimensional echocardiogram with doppler and color flow mapping can identify the absence of blood flow across the pulmonary valve and is diagnostic.

14. All of the following are correct about the treatment of pulmonary atresia in infants EXCEPT: 14.___
   A. Prostaglandin E_1 is used to maintain patency of the ductus arteriosus until surgical intervention.
   B. In most medical centers, a systemic-to-pulmonary shunt such as the Blalock-Taussing operation is performed through a lateral thoracotomy incision.
   C. Some institutions perform a pulmonary valvulotomy or a pulmonary outflow patch procedure.
   D. Both pulmonary valvulotomy and pulmonary outflow patch procedures are performed through a lateral thoracotomy incision.

15. Total anomalous pulmonary venous return (TAPVR) in the neonate is characterized by all the pulmonary veins returning directly or indirectly into the ______, rather than the left atrium. 15.___
   A. right ventricle
   B. left ventricle
   C. right atrium
   D. right atrium and ventricle

16. Neonates with unobstructed TAPVR 16.___
   I. are typically cyanotic
   II. usually have heart murmurs
   III. usually show signs of congestive heart failure resulting from volume overload of the right ventricle
   IV. generally do not demonstrate evidence of congestive heart failure but typically demonstrate pulmonary venous congestion

   The CORRECT answer is:
   A. I, II B. I, III
   C. II, IV D. I, II, III, IV

17. Which of the following is NOT an appropriate laboratory finding in infants with TAPVR? 17.___
   A. The pH and $PaCO_2$ are usually normal. The PaO_2 is mostly high.

B. In obstructed TAPVR, the chest x-ray will show pulmonary venous congestion without cardiomegaly. In unobstructed TAPVR, the chest x-ray will show a marked increase in pulmonary vascularity and cardiomegaly.
C. An electrocardiogram may show right axis deviation, right ventricular hypertrophy, and right atrial enlargement.
D. An echocardiogram is diagnostic. With color flow mapping, the right-to-left shunting across the atrial septum as well as the anomalous venous return can be visualized.

18. All of the following are correct about the treatment of TAPVR EXCEPT: 18.___
A. Unobstructed TAPVR may be medically treated temporarily. Obstructed TAPVR is a surgical emergency.
B. Supracardiac and infracardiac varieties require surgical reimplantation of the common vein into the left atrium.
C. Intracardiac TAPVR can usually be surgically repaired by realigning the atrial septum during closure of the ASD and directing the anomalous veins to the left atrial side.
D. All repairs are performed through a lateral thoracotomy incision.

19. In tricuspid atresia, there is complete agenesis of the tricuspid valve with no direct communication between the right 19.___
A. atrium and right ventricle
B. and left atriums
C. and left ventricles
D. atrium and left ventricle

20. While assessing the infant with tricuspid atresia, all of the following are expected to be noticed EXCEPT 20.___
A. marked cyanosis if the pulmonary blood flow is compromised
B. a double S_2 in infants with tricuspid atresia
C. heart murmurs of associated VSD and PDA shunts
D. congestive heart failure present with a large PDA or VSD shunt

21. Which of the following is NOT an appropriate laboratory finding in the infant with tricuspid atresia? 21.___
A. The pH and $PaCO_2$ are usually elevated. The PaO_2 may vary from near normal, if there is a large VSD or PDA, to extremely low, if there is limited shunting into the pulmonary system.
B. A chest x-ray may show a normal heart size or cardiomegaly. Pulmonary vascularity may be normal, decreased, or increased, depending on the degree of pulmonary blood flow.

C. An electrocardiogram is highly suggestive and usually shows left axis deviation with a counterclockwise loop, a superior axis in the frontal plane, and left ventricular hypertrophy.

D. Absence of the tricuspid valve and presence of a small hypoplastic right ventricle echocardiographically is highly suggestive of tricuspid atresia. Color flow mapping can identify the right-to-left shunt at the atrial level and the presence of a VSD and/or PDA.

22. Regarding the treatment of tricuspid atresia in neonates, it is TRUE that 22.___

I. definitive repair is performed through a lateral thoracotomy incision

II. closure of the ASD and any VSD's present is performed

III. definitive repair of tricuspid atresia involves the creation of a communication between the right atrium and pulmonary artery or right ventricular outflow chamber by direct anastomosis or conduit

IV. when surgery is indicated, the preferred procedure in the neonatal period is a systemic-to-pulmonary shunt such as the Blalock-Taussing operation performed through a lateral thoracotomy incision

The CORRECT answer is:

A. I, III
B. I, II, III
C. I, III, IV
D. II, III, IV

23. An infant with hypertension must be assumed to have a specific secondary etiology. 23.___
All of the following are causes of hypertension in infants EXCEPT

A. hyperplastic abdominal aorta and coarctation of the aorta
B. renal failure and glomerulonephritis
C. adrenogenital syndrome and Cushing's disease
D. bronchopulmonary dysplasia and seizures

24. Which of the following is NOT correct about the signs and symptoms of hypertension in infants? 24.___

A. Any infant exceeding the 95th percentile for blood pressure is considered to be hypertensive.
B. For the term infant, any blood pressure exceeding 95 mmHg systolic or 75 mmHg diastolic is considered hypertensive.
C. Hypertension usually occurs within the first 24 hours of life in the full-term infant and in the fourth week in preterms.
D. Hypertension presents with respiratory distress in 50% of infants; patent ductus arteriosus in 50%; neurologic symptoms such as seizures, tremors, and abnormalities in tone in 30%; and congestive heart failure in 40%.

25. All of the following are true about the treatment of hypertension in the neonate EXCEPT: 25.___
   A. A definable cause, such as a urinary tract obstruction, a tumor, or a coarctation, should be treated surgically
   B. Captopril should be used with caution if there is possible unilateral renal artery stenosis because renal vein thrombosis has been reported in these cases
   C. For an acute hypertensive crisis, IV hydralozine, IV diazoxide, enalapril, and oral captopril are the drugs of choice
   D. Calcium channel blockers have great potential for the treatment of neonatal hypertension

---

KEY (CORRECT ANSWERS)

1. C
2. A
3. D
4. B
5. C

6. B
7. D
8. A
9. C
10. D

11. C
12. C
13. A
14. D
15. C

16. B
17. A
18. D
19. A
20. B

21. A
22. D
23. A
24. C
25. B

TEST 2

DIRECTIONS: Each question or incomplete statement is followed by several suggested answers or completions. Select the one that BEST answers the question or completes the statement. *PRINT THE LETTER OF THE CORRECT ANSWER IN THE SPACE AT THE RIGHT.*

1. Truncus arteriosus in neonates is characterized by one great _____ arising from the _____ ventricle(s) overriding a(n) _____. 1.___
   A. artery; left; PDA
   B. artery; right; ASD
   C. vein; left; PDA
   D. artery; left and right; VSD

2. Assessment findings in the neonate with truncus arteriosus include all of the following EXCEPT: 2.___
   A. The common trunk receives a mixture of unoxygenated blood from the right ventricle and oxygenated blood from the left ventricle
   B. Cyanosis is present at birth but varies in intensity according to the amount of pulmonary blood flow
   C. The first heart sound, S_1, is absent and the S_2 is heard single and loud because of the single valve of the common trunk
   D. Congestive heart failure may be present shortly after birth or appear between 2 and 3 weeks of age

3. Which of the following is NOT a correct laboratory finding in the neonate with truncus arteriosus? 3.___
   A. The pH and $PaCO_2$ are usually normal. If there is no obstruction to pulmonary blood flow, the PaO_2 is normal.
   B. Cardiomegaly, displaced pulmonary arteries, and increased vascular markings are typical findings on the chest x-ray.
   C. Combined ventricular hypertrophy is most often seen in an electrocardiogram. Left atrial enlargement is also commonly found.
   D. The echocardiogram is used to identify the number of truncal valve leaflets, the presence of truncal valve insufficiency, and the presence of pulmonary stenosis.

4. In the treatment of truncus arteriosus in neonates, 4.___
   A. total surgical repair is recommended to be performed in the newborn period
   B. medical management consists of stabilizing and treating congestive heart failure when present. Calcium should be closely monitored because of the possibility of DiGeorge syndrome.
   C. total surgical repair consists of separating the pulmonary vein from the common trunk, closing the ASD with a patch, and inserting a left ventricular-to-pulmonary artery valved conduit
   D. all of the above

5. Hypoplastic left heart syndrome is represented by severe 5.___
   A. coarctation of the aorta
   B. aortic valve stenosis or atresia
   C. mitral valve stenosis or atresia
   D. all of the above

6. Assessment findings in neonates with hypoplastic left heart syndrome include all of the following EXCEPT: 6.___
   A. The infants are mostly severely cyanotic and have severe pallor and a grayish skin color
   B. A nonspecific systolic heart murmur is heard in approximately two-thirds of the infants
   C. Congestive heart failure is present in all cases as a result of right ventricular volume overload
   D. Congestive heart failure is present in all cases as a result of right ventricular pressure overload

7. Which of the following is an INAPPROPRIATE laboratory finding in hypoplastic left heart syndrome of the neonate? 7.___
   A. The arterial blood gases are typically normal until the infant begins to deteriorate.
   B. Cardiomegaly with decreased pulmonary vascularity and pulmonary edema is seen on the chest x-ray.
   C. An electrocardiogram frequently demonstrates right axis deviation and right ventricular hypertrophy; however, electrocardiogram may be normal.
   D. An echocardiogram is usually diagnostic with a small left ventricular cavity and ascending aorta with an abnormal aortic valve pattern.

8. Which of the following is NOT true of the treatment of hypoplastic left heart syndrome in neonates? 8.___
   A. Surgical intervention offers the only chance of neonatal survival. Patency of the ductus arteriosus is maintained with infusion of PGE until surgical intervention.
   B. The initial Norwood procedure consists of enlargement of the atrial septal defect, ligation of the patent ductus arteriosus, anastomosis of the pulmonary artery to the ascending aorta and the aortic arch, and creation of an aorto-pulmonary shunt to maintain pulmonary blood flow.
   C. In the second stage, the aorto-pulmonary shunt is removed and an anastomosis is made between the superior vena cava and the pulmonary artery, which is called the bidirectional Glenn shunt and is performed at 6 to 12 months of age.
   D. The final stage is the Fontan procedure, at 48 to 72 months of age.

9. Premature ventricular beats, brief episodes of ectopic atrial rhythms, wandering atrial pacemakers, and even brief episodes of sinus arrest are all frequently seen in the newborn period. The majority of these dysrhythmias do not require immediate treatment. However, if they persist, all of the following are to be considered EXCEPT 9.____
   A. congenital heart disease and sepsis
   B. drug toxicity and persistent hypoxia
   C. hyperglycemia and hypercalcemia
   D. disorders of electrolyte and acid-base balance

10. Drug therapy for dysrhythmias is based on the ability of certain medications to alter the electrophysiologic properties of cardiac tissue. Of the following drugs, the ones used for the therapy of dysrhythmias in neonates are 10.____
   A. quinidine and lidocaine
   B. procainamide and propranolol
   C. phenytoin and digoxin
   D. all of the above

11. Which of the following are considered to be criteria for supraventricular tachycardia? 11.____
   A. Persistent ventricular rate over 200 beats/minute
   B. A fixed and regular R-R interval
   C. Little change in heart rate with various activities
   D. All of the above

12. Treatment of supraventricular tachycardia in the neonate includes all of the following EXCEPT 12.____
   A. vagal maneuvers, i.e., unilateral carotid pressure, gagging, and rectal stimulation, are found to have very good results
   B. ocular compression should never be used. Overdrive atrial pacing has been successful in converting SVT to normal sinus rhythm
   C. adenosine, a purinergic agonist, is an especially effective antidysrhythmic drug for treatment of SVT
   D. direct-current (DC) cardioversion of 1-2 watt sec/kg is the most effective mode of treatment

13. The presence of atrial flutter and fibrillation in neonates usually indicates severe organic heart disease. Atrial flutter and fibrillation is diagnosed when 13.____
   A. the atrial rate is greater than 220 beats/minute
   B. the P waves are very regular
   C. there is a characteristic sawtooth pattern
   D. all of the above

14. The APPROPRIATE treatment of atrial flutter and fibrillation in neonates is 14.___
   A. DC cardioversion
   B. overdrive atrial pacing
   C. DC cardioversion and overdrive atrial pacing
   D. DC cardioversion or overdrive atrial pacing followed by maintenance therapy with digoxin

15. All of the following are signs and symptoms of acute renal failure in infants EXCEPT: 15.___
   A. ARF presents earlier in the term infant and is more likely to be oliguric
   B. ARF in its nonoliguric form predominates in the postterm infant
   C. Oliguric renal failure includes a urine flow rate of less than 1 ml/kg/hour after the first 48 hours of life
   D. Nonoliguric forms of ARF have a normal urine flow rate with an increase in creatinine

16. Regarding the treatment of acute renal failure in infants, it is TRUE that: 16.___
   I. Prerenal causes require increasing perfusion of the kidney by fluid therapy and restoring cardiac output and blood pressure to normal
   II. A fluid challenge of 20 to 30 ml/kg of body weight of colloid should be attempted. These fluids may exacerbate lung disease or heart failure and should be administered with caution.
   III. Aggressive therapy of any infections is important because sepsis can be fatal in the neonate with renal failure
   IV. Dialysis should be used only when complications of ARF are no longer medically manageable

   The CORRECT answer is:
   A. I, II
   B. I, II, III
   C. I, III, IV
   D. II, III, IV

17. Polycystic kidney disease (PKD) may present as one of two types in the infant: (1) infantile type (ICPD), which is autosomal recessive, or (2) adult type, which is autosomal dominant. 17.___
   Criteria for making a definitive diagnosis for both diseases include all of the following EXCEPT
   A. congenital hepatic fibrosis on liver biopsy or evidence of portal hypertension
   B. renal histologic studies consistent with renal vein ectopia
   C. positive parental history
   D. known liver cysts or Berry aneurysm

18. The signs and symptoms of polycystic kidney disease of both types in infants do NOT include 18.___
   A. hypertension
   B. hyperplastic lungs
   C. Potter's facies caused by oligohydramnios
   D. respiratory distress

19. Neonates with either form of polycystic kidney disease need 19.___
   A. aggressive treatment of blood pressure with captopril as the drug of choice
   B. treatment of any urinary tract infection
   C. aggressive nutritional management, including a protein-restricted diet
   D. all of the above

20. All of the following provide appropriate information about hydronephrosis in infants EXCEPT: 20.___
   A. Hydronephrosis involves a dilation of the pelvis and calyces, most often as a result of congenital obstruction. The most common ureteral site of obstruction is the ureteropelvic junction.
   B. Posterior urethral valves in males are the major causes of urethral obstruction. This distal obstruction may result in bladder hypertrophy, hydroureter, and hydronephrosis if severe.
   C. A viable fetus with dilated collecting systems, initial normal amount of amniotic fluid, and evidence of decreasing amniotic fluid should be delivered early
   D. The surgical correction of obstruction at the uteropelvic and/or uterovesical junctions is contraindicated

21. Renal vein thrombosis (RVT) in infants is associated with conditions that cause circulatory collapse and decreased oxygenation within the kidney. 21.___
Perinatal causes of neonatal RVT include all of the following EXCEPT
   A. maternal diabetes
   B. placental insufficiency
   C. postmaturity
   D. respiratory distress syndrome

22. The signs and symptoms of renal vein thrombosis in infants do NOT include 22.___
   A. thrombocytopenia and acute renal failure
   B. hematuria in about 60% of cases
   C. anemia and oliguria
   D. the involved kidney engorging with blood because of obstruction to blood flow and forming a palpable flank mass

23. The treatment of renal vein thrombosis in infants includes all of the following EXCEPT: 23.___
   A. Management includes treatment of the underlying illness, treatment of sepsis if suspected, fluid therapy, and possibly dialysis in select cases
   B. Heparin therapy has been used most successfully
   C. Rarely nephrectomy is required
   D. Surgical excision of the thrombus is not usually indicated during the acute phase but may be appropriate at a later time

24. Which of the following does NOT provide correct information about urinary tract infections in infants? 24.___
   A. UTI's affect approximately 1% of full-term infants and 3% of premature infants. Male infants are affected 5 times more frequently than females.
   B. Symptomatic manifestations include abnormal weight loss during the first days of life, dehydration, lethargy, irritability, cyanosis, jaundice, and septicemia. Infected infants may also be asymptomatic.
   C. The optimum method of obtaining urine for culture is a suprapubic aspiration of the bladder.
   D. Grades of reflux are diagnosed by VCUG. Successful urine test results depend on an empty bladder.

25. All of the following statements about the treatment of urinary tract infection in infants are correct EXCEPT: 25.___
   A. Pyuria 10 to 15 WBC/hpf can be observed in the neonate normally. Treatment for UTI is indicated when an organism is cultured from the urine.
   B. Traditional antibiotic coverage consists of both ampicillin and an aminoglycoside. Cephalosporins provide excellent gram-negative coverage without the nephrotoxicity of the aminoglycosides.
   C. Sulfonamides are recommended in the neonate because of their potential to correct hyperbilirubinemia
   D. Antibiotic therapy should continue for 14 days, with a follow-up urine culture 3 days after the therapy is over

KEY (CORRECT ANSWERS)

1. D	6. A	11. D	16. C	21. C
2. C	7. B	12. A	17. B	22. A
3. A	8. D	13. D	18. B	23. B
4. B	9. C	14. D	19. D	24. D
5. D	10. D	15. B	20. D	25. C

EXAMINATION SECTION
TEST 1

DIRECTIONS: Each question or incomplete statement is followed by several suggested answers or completions. Select the one that BEST answers the question or completes the statement. *PRINT THE LETTER OF THE CORRECT ANSWER IN THE SPACE AT THE RIGHT.*

1. The most serious of the postnatal infections is sepsis. All of the following are common organisms known to cause early-onset bacterial sepsis EXCEPT 1.___
   A. Group B streptococcus
   B. Escherichia coli
   C. haemophilus influenzae, type B and nontypable
   D. Klebsiella pneumoniae

2. Bacteria responsible for early-onset bacterial sepsis in the neonate are acquired before delivery from 2.___
   A. the birth canal
   B. human contact
   C. the maternal genital tract
   D. contaminated equipment or material

3. Bacteria responsible for late-onset sepsis and meningitis in the neonate include those acquired from all of the following EXCEPT 3.___
   A. the maternal genital tract
   B. human contact
   C. the birth canal
   D. contaminated equipment or material

4. Hand washing is the most important procedure for controlling infection in the NICU. Which of the following practices is NOT considered to be an appropriate hand washing principle? 4.___
   A. Before each shift wash hands, wrists, forearms, and elbows with an antiseptic.
   B. Wash hands for 10-15 seconds between infant contacts.
   C. Soap and water are adequate for hand washing unless the infant is infected or contaminated objects have been handled.
   D. Wash hands with medicated soap and sterilized water before surgical or similar invasive procedures.

5. In general, signs, particularly of early-onset bacterial sepsis, are nonspecific and nonlocalizing. Assessment findings include: 5.___
   I. Stable temperature
   II. Lethargy and jaundice
   III. Seizures and respiratory distress
   IV. Purpura and opthalmia neonatorum

The CORRECT answer is:
A. I, II
B. I, II, IV
C. II, III
D. III, IV

6. Isolating bacteria from the _____ is NOT one of the most valid methods of establishing the diagnosis of bacterial sepsis in the neonate. 6.___
A. blood
B. saliva
C. urine
D. CSF

7. One of the MOST common complications of bacterial sepsis in neonates is 7.___
A. proctitis
B. cellulitis
C. pyomyositis
D. meningitis

8. All of the following infants are at increased risk for fungal infection EXCEPT those 8.___
A. requiring surgery
B. requiring invasive procedures such as arterial or venous catheters
C. with very high birth weight
D. none of the above

9. Because of the movement of lung fluid and its components, notably lecithin, into amniotic fluid, the lecithin/sphingomyelin (L/S) ratio has become a notable clinical tool for predicting infants at risk for respiratory distress syndrome (RDS). 9.___
In general, the L/S ratio associated with RDS is
A. more than 2:1
B. less than 2:1
C. more than 3:1
D. less than 3:1

10. All of the following are the true characteristics of respiratory distress syndrome (RDS) in the neonate EXCEPT: 10.___
A. Prematurity is the single most common factor in the occurrence of RDS
B. Its incidence is inversely proportional to gestational age and occurs most frequently in infants of less than 1200 g and 30 weeks' gestation
C. Affected female infants outnumber affected male infants 2:1
D. The principal factor operating in the development of RDS in very premature infants is surfactant deficiency

11. When the neonate is unable to maintain adequate oxygenation because of a respiratory disease, supplemental oxygen must be provided. 11.___
To prevent respiratory therapy equipment from becoming a source of infection, humidifiers and tubing should be replaced AT LEAST every _____ hours.
A. 12
B. 24
C. 36
D. 48

12. Whenever the normal mechanisms for mobilizing and removing pulmonary secretions are inefficient or inactive, pulmonary hygiene is indicated. 12.___
Which of the following is NOT one of the goals of pulmonary hygiene?
To
A. facilitate removal of pulmonary debris by loosening and mobilizing secretions into the mainstem bronchi for suctioning
B. maintain a patent airway
C. prevent excessive pulmonary ventilation
D. prevent pulmonary infection from accumulated secretions

13. In a pulmonary disease of the neonate, chest physiotherapy may be indicated by the physician due to respiratory distress. 13.___
Chest physiotherapy consists of
I. positioning
II. percussion
III. vibration
IV. suction

The CORRECT answer is:
A. II *only*
B. III,IV
C. II, III
D. I, II, III

14. In a respiratory disease, acute and chronic complications are the result of the disease process or treatment, or both. 14.___
Acute complications of respiratory diseases in the neonate do NOT include
A. hypoxic-ischemic injury
B. oxygen toxicity and barotrauma (BPD)
C. bleeding diathesis
D. decreased cardiac output

15. Pneumothorax or other air leaks should be suspected when any one of the following infants takes a sudden turn for the worse EXCEPT a(n) 15.___
A. preterm infant with RDS either with or without positive-pressure support
B. term or postterm infant with meconium-stained amniotic fluid
C. infant with an x-ray picture of interstitial or labor emphysema
D. infant requiring resuscitation 48 to 96 hours after birth

16. A suggested conservative treatment of the affected lung in an air leak problem of the neonate is 16.___
A. bronchodilatation
B. endotracheal intubation
C. surfactant replacement therapy
D. medications blocking histamine release

17. All of the following are signs and symptoms of bronchopulmonary dysplasia, known as one of the most serious chronic complications of the neonatal respiratory diseases, EXCEPT 17.___
   A. cardiomyopathy
   B. exercise intolerance
   C. oxygen dependence
   D. respiratory distress

18. Complications of bronchopulmonary dysplasia do NOT include 18.___
   A. progressive interstitial emphysema and cyst formation; air leaks
   B. pulmonary hypertension; cor-pulmonale
   C. bronchiolitis most common between 2 to 4 years of age
   D. fractures from vigorous chest physiotherapy; rickets

19. Which of the following factors contribute to the development of retinopathy of prematurity (ROP)? 19.___
   I. Hypercapnia or hypocapnia; multiple gestation
   II. Asphyxia; sepsis
   III. Blood transfusions; apnea
   IV. Birth weight less than 2500; hyperoxia

   The CORRECT answer is:
   A. I, II, III
   B. I, II, IV
   C. II, III, IV
   D. III, IV

20. Transient tachypnea of the newborn GENERALLY occurs in _____ babies. 20.___
   A. term or near-term
   B. preterm
   C. postterm
   D. all of the above

21. The laboratory data of an infant with transient tachypnea of the newborn USUALLY shows the presence of 21.___
   A. severe hypoxemia
   B. severe acidemia
   C. severe hypoxemia and severe acidemia
   D. mild hypoxemia and mild acidemia

22. Laboratory findings in the neonate with meconium aspiration do NOT usually include severe 22.___
   A. hypoxemia
   B. hypotension
   C. hypercapnia
   D. acidosis

23. Risk factors of persistent pulmonary hypertension of the newborn (PPHN), a frequent complication of meconium aspiration, include all of the following EXCEPT 23.___
   A. fetal hypertension and pulmonary hypoplasia
   B. polycythemia and hypothermia
   C. myocardial dysfunction and ischemia and sepsis
   D. alveolar hyperventilation and pneumonia

24. All of the following are common radiographic findings associated with persistent pulmonary hypertension of the newborn EXCEPT 24.___
   A. prominent pulmonary vein segment
   B. mild-to-moderate cardiomegaly
   C. variable pulmonary vasculature
   D. signs of left ventricular dysfunction that include pulmonary venous congestion and cardiomegaly

25. Cyanosis in the neonate is a bluish discoloration of the skin, nail beds, and mucous membranes resulting from the presence of ______ blood. 25.___
   A. 3 mg/dl or more of reduced hemoglobin in the arterial
   B. 4 to 5 mg/dl or more of reduced hemoglobin in the peripheral capillary
   C. reduced hemoglobin in both the arterial and peripheral capillary
   D. none of the above

KEY (CORRECT ANSWERS)

1. D
2. A
3. C
4. D
5. C

6. B
7. D
8. C
9. B
10. C

11. D
12. C
13. D
14. B
15. D

16. B
17. A
18. C
19. A
20. A

21. D
22. B
23. D
24. A
25. C

TEST 2

DIRECTIONS: Each question or incomplete statement is followed by several suggested answers or completions. Select the one that BEST answers the question or completes the statement. *PRINT THE LETTER OF THE CORRECT ANSWER IN THE SPACE AT THE RIGHT.*

1. Iatrogenic causes of neonatal apnea do NOT include 1.___
   A. sudden increases in environmental temperature
   B. nasopharyngeal reflux
   C. obstruction of the airway
   D. vagal response to suctioning of the nasopharynx or to a gavage tube

2. All of the following are appropriate measures used for the prevention of apnea in neonates EXCEPT: 2.___
   A. All infants assessed as high risk for apneic spells should be carefully monitored for a period of at least 4 to 6 days
   B. Pulse oximetry or $TcPO_2$ monitors may detect hypoxemic conditions that may lead to apneic spells
   C. Gentle tactile stimulation alone has been shown to be effective in decreasing and preventing apneic spells in most premature infants
   D. Careful attention must be paid to prevent airway obstruction

3. Which of the following shunts allows mixing of the fetal blood and is important in the development of a normal heart? 3.___
   A. Ductus arteriosus B. Ductus venosus
   C. Foramen ovale D. All of the above

4. Newborns with severe congenital heart disease may have the following signs or symptoms: 4.___
   I. Respiratory distress and angina pectoris
   II. Congestive heart failure and diminished cardiac output
   III. Cyanosis and myocardial infarction
   IV. Abnormal cardiac rhythm and cardiac murmurs

   The CORRECT answer is:
   A. I, II B. I, III
   C. II, IV D. III, IV

5. Congestive heart failure is a clinical syndrome reflecting the inability of the myocardium to meet the metabolic requirements of the body. 5.___
   Congestive heart failure in the newborn may be caused by all of the following EXCEPT
   A. asphyxia and anemia
   B. volume overload and pressure overload
   C. cardiomyopathy and dysrhythmias
   D. cyanosis and increased left atrial/aortic ratio

6. The expected laboratory findings in neonatal patent ductus arteriosus do NOT include 6.___
   A. abnormal arterial blood gases
   B. normal chest x-ray in small shunts; cardiomegaly present with increased pulmonary vascularity in large shunts
   C. electrocardiogram may be normal, demonstrate left ventricular hypertrophy, or demonstrate combined ventricular hypertrophy; ischemia is rarely seen
   D. echocardiogram showing an increased left atrial/aortic ratio suggests a moderate to large left to right shunt

7. Asymptomatic infants with patent ductus arteriosus (PDS) generally do not require medical management or surgical ligation. Symptomatic infants require ductal closure by either ductal ligation or indomethacin therapy. Indomethacin is administered orally (PO) or intravenously (IV) at _____ mg/kg/dose and may be repeated every 8 hours for a total of three doses. 7.___
   A. 0.1 to 0.2
   B. 1 to 2
   C. 2 to 3
   D. 3 to 4

8. Which of the following is an INCORRECT laboratory finding in ventricular septal defect (VSD) of the neonate? 8.___
   A. Arterial blood gases are normal.
   B. The chest x-ray shows a normal to increased heart size with an increased pulmonary vascular flow.
   C. The electrocardiogram is mostly abnormal showing ventricular atrophy.
   D. A two-dimensional echocardiogram is able to demonstrate the VSD's in 90% of the cases.

9. All of the following are correct statements regarding surgical treatment of ventricular septal defects (VSD's) in neonates EXCEPT: 9.___
   A. Surgical treatment of a VSD consists of either suture closure or patching
   B. If the infant weighs 2 to 4 kg, it is necessary to perform a palliative procedure of pulmonary artery banding to decrease pulmonary blood flow until the infant is older and can undergo debanding and closure of the VSD's
   C. In general, a VSD may be approached through a median sternotomy incision, then through the right atrium and tricuspid valve, thereby avoiding a right or left ventriculotomy
   D. Suture closure or patching is performed using, most commonly, a synthetic material such as Dacron

10. In the neonates, coarctation of the aorta is a localized constriction of the aorta that can occur anywhere in the aorta from _____ to the abdominal aorta. 10.___
   A. above the transverse aortic arch
   B. below the descending aorta
   C. above the ascending aorta
   D. above the aortic valve

11. Coarctation is frequently observed in infants with _____ syndrome. 11.___
   A. Down's
   B. Kawasaki
   C. Marfan
   D. Turner's

12. All of the following are correct laboratory findings in coarctation of the aorta in the neonate EXCEPT: 12.___
   A. Arterial blood gases are normal
   B. In chest x-ray, pulmonary vascularity is always normal but cardiomegaly may be seen
   C. In electrocardiogram, right ventricular hypertrophy is frequently seen. Left ventricular hypertrophy or combined ventricular hypertrophy is rarely seen in the newborn period
   D. Using two-dimensional echocardiogram and color flow mapping, the area of coarctation can often be visualized. Abnormal Doppler blood flow is diagnostic.

13. Intractable congestive heart failure, acidosis, oliguria, and hypertension are indications for corrective surgery in coarctation of the aorta in the neonates. 13.___
The two MOST common surgical procedures are
   A. suture closures and resection of the coarctation with end-to-end anostomosis
   B. patching and subclavian flap aortoplasty
   C. aortic valvulotomy and patching
   D. resection of the coarctation with end-to-end anostomosis and subclavian flap aortoplasty

14. A pressure difference from the left ventricle to the ascending aorta of 50 mm Hg or more is indicative of significant aortic stenosis in the newborn. 14.___
All of the following are correct assessment findings in an infant with aortic stenosis EXCEPT
   A. pale, gray, cool skin with decreased perfusion and peripheral pulses
   B. cyanosis is mostly present in isolated valvular aortic stenosis
   C. a grade II to IV/VI harsh systolic murmur in the upper right sternal border, radiating to the upper left sternal border and faintly to the neck
   D. with critical aortic stenosis, congestive heart failure caused by a pressure overload of the left ventricle

15. Which of the following is NOT an appropriate laboratory finding for the neonate with critical aortic stenosis? 15.___
   A. Usually altered arterial blood gases
   B. Chest x-ray shows cardiomegaly with normal pulmonary vascularity
   C. Electrocardiogram may be normal or demonstrate left ventricular hypertrophy
   D. Aortic valve is usually thickened and appears to close abnormally on an echocardiogram

16. Medical management is usually unsatisfactory, and surgical intervention is necessary for critical aortic stenosis in the newborn. 16.___
The surgical procedure MOST often used for correcting aortic stenosis in infants is
   A. subclavian flap aortoplasty
   B. patching
   C. surgical ligation through a lateral thoracotomy incision
   D. aortic volvulotomy through a median sternotomy incision

17. In critical pulmonary stenosis with intact ventricular septum, the flow to the pulmonary artery from the right ventricle is obstructed. 17.___
All of the following are correct assessment findings in infants with critical pulmonary stenosis EXCEPT:
   A. Cyanosis is generally not present in an isolated lesion but may occur in the presence of a right-to-left atrial shunt
   B. A harsh, grade II to III/VI systolic murmur is heard in the upper left sternal border, radiating to both axillae and faintly to the back
   C. A murmur of bicuspid insufficiency is heard
   D. The infant with critical pulmonary stenosis typically has signs and symptoms of right-sided congestive heart failure resulting from excessive pressure overload

18. It is NOT true, regarding appropriate laboratory findings in infants with critical pulmonary stenosis, that 18.___
   A. arterial blood gases are mostly altered
   B. the chest x-ray may be normal but it usually demonstrates cardiomegaly with normal or decreased pulmonary vascularity
   C. the electrocardiogram may be normal or show right ventricular hypertrophy
   D. an abnormal pulmonary valve pattern on a two-dimensional echocardiogram is diagnostic

19. The preferable surgical procedure for the treatment of critical pulmonary stenosis in infants, if the right ventricle and pulmonary arteries are of adequate size, is 19.___
   A. subclavian flap pulmonplasty
   B. suture closure or patching
   C. clipping through a lateral thoracotomy incision
   D. pulmonary valvulotomy through a median sternotomy incision

20. Expected assessment findings in infants with atrioventricular septal defect include: 20.___
   I. Generally, cyanosis is not present with an isolated endocardial cushion defect
   II. If tricuspid insufficiency is present, a blowing, diastolic, apical murmur with radiation to the right axilla and/or a VSD murmur is heard
   III. If mitral insufficiency is present, a blowing, systolic, apical murmur with radiation to the left axilla and/or a VSD murmur is heard
   IV. Congestive heart failure may be present because of volume overload of the ventricles as a result of mitral insufficiency and left-to-right shunting at either the atrial or ventricular level

   The CORRECT answer is:
   A. I, II B. I, II, III
   C. I, III, IV D. II, III, IV

21. Which of the following is NOT an appropriate laboratory finding in infants with atrioventricular septal defect? 21.___
   A. The $PaCO_2$ may be elevated if there is a severe mitral insufficiency and pulmonary edema. The pH and PaO_2 are usually normal.
   B. In chest x-ray, the heart size may be normal or increased. Pulmonary vascularity is mostly decreased.
   C. An electrocardiogram with a left axis deviation, counterclockwise loop in the frontal plane, and superior axis suggests AV septal defect.
   D. A two-dimensional echocardiogram with doppler and color flow mapping demonstrates the ASD, VSD, and common AV valves, and the degree of AV valve insufficiency. This technique is diagnostic.

22. The surgical treatment of an infant with AV septal defect through a median sternotomy incision involves 22.___
   A. closing the ASD and VSD
   B. separating the common leaflets of the mitral and tricuspid valves
   C. reconstructing the mitral valve
   D. all of the above

23. Infants with abnormally elevated pulmonary vascular resistance have persistent pulmonary hypertension of the newborn.
The assessment findings in this case include all of the following EXCEPT 23.___
   A. milder cases have minimal transient tachycardia associated with hypoxia
   B. severe cases have marked cyanosis, tachypnea, acidosis, and decreased peripheral perfusion
   C. a loud pulmonary component of S_2 and occasionally a nonspecific systolic ejection murmur are heard
   D. congestive heart failure is usually present because of pressure overload of the right ventricle

24. Of the following, the INAPPROPRIATE laboratory finding in infants with persistent pulmonary hypertension is: 24.___
   A. Arterial blood gases demonstrate acidosis, hypoxia, and decreased $PaCO_2$
   B. The chest x-ray demonstrates mild to moderate cardiomegaly with normal pulmonary vascularity
   C. The electrocardiogram frequently is normal but may demonstrate right ventricular hypertrophy and signs of myocardial ischemia
   D. An echocardiogram helps to evaluate cardiac structures and rule out cyanotic lesions

25. Which of the following is NOT an appropriate measure used in the treatment of persistent pulmonary hypertension of the newborn? 25.___
   A. Intervention is aimed at using various maneuvers to increase pulmonary blood flow.
   B. The infant should be ventilated with whatever combination of rate, pressure, and oxygen is needed to lower $PaCO_2$ and pH.
   C. In the presence of systemic hypertension, volume expansion with albumin, plasma, or blood is instituted.
   D. Infusion of vasopressors and/or afterload reducers has been advocated.

KEY (CORRECT ANSWERS)

1. B	6. A	11. D	16. D	21. B
2. A	7. A	12. B	17. C	22. D
3. D	8. C	13. D	18. A	23. A
4. C	9. B	14. B	19. D	24. A
5. D	10. D	15. A	20. C	25. C

EXAMINATION SECTION
TEST 1

DIRECTIONS: Each question or incomplete statement is followed by several suggested answers or completions. Select the one that BEST answers the question or completes the statement. *PRINT THE LETTER OF THE CORRECT ANSWER IN THE SPACE AT THE RIGHT.*

1. All of the following criteria rule out the diagnosis of physiologic jaundice EXCEPT 1.___
   A. clinical jaundice in the first 72 hours of life
   B. total serum bilirubin concentration exceeding 12.9 mg/dl in a full-term infant or 15 mg/dl in a premature infant
   C. direct serum bilirubin concentration exceeding 1.5 to 2 mg/dl
   D. clinical jaundice persisting for more than 1 week in a full-term infant or 2 weeks in a premature infant

2. The presence of nonglucose-reducing substances in the urine of a neonate suggests 2.___
   A. galactokinosemia
   B. galactorrhea
   C. galactosemia
   D. galactokinase deficiency

3. The widespread use of ______ in IDM has proved effective in preventing the sensitization of RH-negative mothers after delivery or abortion of RH-positive infants. 3.___
   A. gamma aminobutyric acid
   B. IgD
   C. anti-D gamma globulin (RhoGAM)
   D. IgA

4. Phenobarbital acts as an inducer of microsomal enzymes, increasing the conjugation of bilirubin. Which of the following is CORRECT about the use of phenobarbital? 4.___
   A. It is effective when given to the mother before delivery.
   B. In infants with significant hemolytic disease of the newborn, it appears to slow the rate of rise of bilirubin and decrease the incidence of exchange transfusion.
   C. It is indicated in infants with Crigler-Najjar syndrome type II.
   D. All of the above

5. Recent clinical trials have shown that tin protoporphyrin (SnPP) decreases bilirubin production when given to infants with 5.___
   A. polycythemia
   B. breast milk jaundice
   C. breastfeeding jaundice
   D. ABO hemolytic disease

6. The assessment of a jaundiced infant may show the occurrence of all of the following signs and symptoms EXCEPT: 6.____
   A. In the absence of hemolysis, an infant may be symptomatic with dermal icterus as the only clinical sign
   B. The infant with hemolytic disease of the newborn may show signs of jaundice and pallor in association with severe anemia and hydrops fetalis or may appear entirely normal at birth
   C. Hepatosplenomegaly resulting from congestion and extramedullary hemopoiesis may be present
   D. The presence of petechiae or purpura raises the possibility of intrauterine infection or sepsis

7. Which of the following is NOT a correct laboratory finding for a jaundiced infant? 7.____
   A. Coombs' test on cord blood is positive in ABO disease. Later testing of the infant's blood in an ABO incompatibility may be Coombs' negative.
   B. A careful examination of the peripheral blood smear may show evidence of hemolysis, such as increased number of nucleated RBCs or the presence of fragmented cells, poikilocytosis, and anisocytosis.
   C. Spherocytosis is characteristic of ABO incompatibility and may at times be confused with hereditary microspherocytosis.
   D. An abnormal white blood cell count or differential or thrombocytopenia may suggest infection.

8. Jaundice in the newborn can usually be detected clinically at a level of _____ mg/dl. 8.____
   A. 2 to 3 B. 6 to 7 C. 12 to 13 D. 20 to 21

9. In the newborn with jaundice, visible icterus appears first on the head and face. 9.____
   The last skin surface to be affected is the
   A. back B. chest
   C. abdomen D. extremities

10. Immediate exchange transfusion with Type _____ RH-_____ red blood cells may be necessary in RH-incompatibility with a severely affected jaundiced infant. 10.____
   A. O; positive B. AB; negative
   C. O; negative D. AB; positive

11. Minimal laboratory evaluation of the jaundiced newborn should include all of the following EXCEPT 11.____
   A. mother's and infant's blood types; RH status
   B. complete blood count; white blood cell count and differential
   C. peripheral smear for red blood cell morphology; hematocrit
   D. Coombs' test on peripheral blood

12. Little evidence of adverse effects of bilirubin on IQ, neurologic examination, or hearing has been found in full-term infants without hemolytic disease. Newman and Maisels have suggested that, in this population of infants, risks of exchange transfusion outweigh benefits until total serum bilirubin is _____ mg/dl. 12.___
   A. 15 to 20 B. 20 to 25 C. 25 to 30 D. 30 to 35

13. In the case of full-term infants without hemolytic disease, a suggested guideline is to initiate phototherapy when the serum bilirubin is below _____ mg/dl of the serum bilirubin concentration at which an exchange transfusion will be performed for that individual infant. 13.___
   A. 5 B. 10 C. 15 D. 20

14. Phototherapy of jaundiced infants generally consists of a single quartz halogen lamp or a bank of four to eight cool white, daybright, or special blue fluorescent bulbs covered by a plexiglas shield and placed from the patient at a distance of _____ inches. 14.___
   A. 8 to 12 B. 12 to 30 C. 8 to 20 D. 6 to 24

15. While performing phototherapy in jaundiced infants, the MOST effective spectrum of light is at _____ nm efficiency. 15.___
   A. 220 to 260
   B. 280 to 340
   C. 360 to 400
   D. 420 to 460

16. In jaundiced infants, administration of 1 g/kg of salt-poor albumin _____ the exchange transfusion has been shown in some studies to increase the efficiency of exchange transfusion by about 40%. 16.___
   A. 1 hour before
   B. together with
   C. just after
   D. 1 hour after

17. The rate of exchange transfusion in jaundiced infants is usually 2 to 4 ml/minute. Blood used in the exchange should be warmed and mixed in the bag after every _____ milliliters. 17.___
   A. 30 to 80 B. 50 to 100 C. 70 to 140 D. 80 to 160

18. While performing exchange transfusion in a jaundiced infant, the infant should be evaluated for hypocalcemia after each _____ ml of the exchange has been completed. 18.___
   A. 50 B. 100 C. 150 D. 200

19. The one of the following that is NOT a known complication of phototherapy is 19.___
   A. increased insensible water loss
   B. loose bowel movements
   C. increased platelet count
   D. bronze baby syndrome

20. Exchange transfusion in jaundiced infants is a procedure with risk for all of the following complications EXCEPT 20.___
   A. thrombosis and necrotizing enterocolitis
   B. thrombocytopenia and bleeding
   C. bacteremia and blood-borne, viral hepatitis
   D. acidosis and hypercalcemia

21. In exchange transfusion of jaundiced infants, heparinized blood must be used within ______ hours of preparation of the unit. 21.___
   A. 6 B. 12 C. 24 D. 48

22. The nurse, while assessing an infant with hepatitis B, may expect to notice all of the following EXCEPT 22.___
   A. the infant is mostly symptomatic
   B. occasionally, infected infant demonstrates elevated liver enzymes
   C. uncommon finding of acute fulminating hepatitis
   D. neonatal infection with subsequent chronic carriage has been implicated in the development of primary hepatocellular carcinoma later in life

23. Virtually what percentage of infants at risk of acquiring hepatitis from their mothers are HBsAg negative at birth? 23.___
   A. 25% B. 50% C. 75% D. 100%

24. An infant with cytomegalovirus (CMV) is usually asymptomatic. 24.___
Congenital manifestations include all of the following EXCEPT
   A. intrauterine growth retardation and neonatal jaundice
   B. hepatosplenomegaly and microcephaly
   C. progressive sensorineural hearing loss and septic joints
   D. brain damage and chorioretinitis

25. While obtaining laboratory data of the infant, CMV may be cultured from 25.___
   A. urine B. pharyngeal secretions
   C. peripheral leukocytes D. all of the above

KEY (CORRECT ANSWERS)

1. A	6. A	11. D	16. A	21. C
2. C	7. C	12. C	17. B	22. A
3. C	8. B	13. A	18. B	23. D
4. D	9. D	14. B	19. C	24. C
5. D	10. C	15. D	20. D	25. D

TEST 2

DIRECTIONS: Each question or incomplete statement is followed by several suggested answers or completions. Select the one that BEST answers the question or completes the statement. *PRINT THE LETTER OF THE CORRECT ANSWER IN THE SPACE AT THE RIGHT.*

1. Epidemiologic evidence has NOT implicated which of the following in transmission of the human immunodeficiency virus (HIV) from mother to the neonate? 1.___
   A. Blood
   B. Vaginal secretions
   C. Saliva
   D. Breast milk

2. Infants with perinatally acquired HIV infection rarely have symptoms in the neonatal period, but the majority of these infants will present with clinical illness by 24 months of life. 2.___
   These symptoms may include all of the following EXCEPT
   A. generalized lymphadenopathy and hepatosplenomegaly
   B. osteomyelitis and pneumonia
   C. sepsis and meningitis
   D. persistent oral candidiasis and chronic or recurrent constipation

3. The PRIMARY serologic laboratory test used to identify HIV in the neonate is the 3.___
   A. polymerase chain reaction test
   B. P24 antigen test
   C. HIV-specific IgA test
   D. enzyme-linked immunosorbent assay (ELISA)

4. Rubella has a high incidence of sequelae in the infant during which period of pregnancy? 4.___
   A. First 3 months
   B. First 4 to 5 months
   C. First 6 months
   D. 6 months to delivery

5. NOT included among the signs and/or symptoms of rubella in the neonate is 5.___
   A. cataracts and neonatal jaundice
   B. hepatosplenomegaly and purpura
   C. chronic encephalitis and microcephaly
   D. cardiac defects and intracerebral calcification

6. In obtaining the laboratory data of an infant with rubella, the virus may be isolated from all of the following EXCEPT the 6.___
   A. peripheral leukocytes
   B. blood and urine
   C. throat
   D. cerebrospinal fluid (CSF)

7. An infant exposed to syphilis may be asymptomatic at birth. 7.____
Neonatal manifestations do NOT include
A. hepatitis and pneumonitis
B. bone marrow failure and nephrotic syndrome
C. myocarditis and meningitis
D. rhinitis and a rash involving the neck and the back

8. All of the following are diagnostic tests for syphilis in the neonate EXCEPT 8.____
A. Venereal Disease Research Laboratory (VDRL) tests
B. rapid plasma reagin (RPR) tests
C. hemagglutination inhibition (IHA) test
D. microhemagglutination test for treponema pallidum (MHA-TP)

9. VDRL tests on the _____ are mandatory in all infants suspected of having congenital syphilis. 9.____
A. peripheral blood
B. cord blood
C. urine
D. CSF

10. Manifestations of toxoplasmosis in the newborn may include all of the following EXCEPT 10.____
A. chorioretinitis and seizures
B. cerebral calcification and hepatosplenomegaly
C. thrombocytopenia and postmaturity
D. generalized lymphadenopathy and jaundice

11. In the infant with toxoplasmosis, the toxoplasma gondii cysts may be found in the 11.____
A. placenta
B. tissues of the fetus
C. tissues of the newborn
D. all of the above

12. A mother with chlamydia trachomatis is usually asymptomatic during her pregnancy. 12.____
All of the following are known signs and symptoms in the infant exposed to chlamydia trachomatis EXCEPT:
A. Conjunctivitis may be manifested as congestion and edema of the conjunctiva with minimal discharge developing 1 to 2 weeks after birth and lasting several weeks with recurrences, particularly after topical therapy
B. Infants with penumonitis mostly reach a fever of 102°F and above with chills
C. Infants with pneumonitis have a prolonged staccato cough, tachypnea, mild hypoxemia, and eosinophilia
D. Otitis media and bronchiolitis may also occur

13. While obtaining laboratory data of an infant exposed to chlamydia trachomatis, scraping conjunctival epithelial cells and demonstrating characteristic intracytoplasmic inclusion bodies by which of the following tests is diagnostic? 13.____
A. Serum antibody tests
B. Serologic tests
C. Direct immunofluorescence
D. A giemsa stain

14. Signs and symptoms in infants exposed to enterovirus may include all of the following EXCEPT: 14.____
    A. Intrauterine growth retardation
    B. Infants may be asymptomatic or have fever or diarrhea
    C. Fulminating encephalomyocarditis may occur within several days of birth
    D. Acute hepatic necrosis may occur within several days of birth

15. Definitive diagnosis in infants exposed to enterovirus CANNOT be made by isolating the organism from the 15.____
    A. throat B. rectum
    C. tissue culture cells D. CFS

16. The key to preventing herpes simplex (types 1 and 2) in infants is avoiding exposure. 16.____
    Mothers with active lesions or prodromes should have cesarean section PREFERABLY within _____ hours of membrane rupture.
    A. 1 to 3 B. 2 to 4 C. 3 to 5 D. 4 to 6

17. Assessment findings of infants with herpes simplex include all of the following EXCEPT 17.____
    A. localized skin lesions
    B. generalized infections involving the liver and lungs
    C. generalized infection of kidneys
    D. generalized infection involving the central nervous system (CNS)

18. In infants with herpes simplex, the virus may be readily identified on a tissue culture, within 24 to 48 hours, from the 18.____
    A. respiratory and genital tracts
    B. blood and urine
    C. CSF
    D. all of the above

19. While obtaining the laboratory data of the infant with mycobacterium tuberculosis, acid-fast organisms found on smears of which of the following STRONGLY suggest tuberculosis in the infant? 19.____
    A. Gastric aspirates and sputum
    B. Infected tissues
    C. CSF
    D. All of the above

20. In gonorrhea-positive mothers, it is mandatory in all vaginal deliveries to administer _____ in the neonate's eyes. 20.____
    A. silver nitrate B. erythromycin
    C. tetracycline D. all of the above

21. The predominant manifestation of gonorrhea in exposed infants is through 21.___
   A. ophthalmia neonatorum
   B. endocardium and CNS infection
   C. scalp abscess
   D. blood-borne infection involving the joints and lungs

22. In an infant exposed to gonorrhea, the laboratory finding of a Gram's stain of purulent eye discharge revealing gram-______ is diagnostic. 22.___
   A. negative anaerobic bacilli
   B. positive intracellular diplococci
   C. negative intracellular diplococci
   D. positive aerobic bacilli

23. Congenital varicella is rare but has followed maternal varicella in the _____ trimester of pregnancy. 23.___
   A. first
   B. second
   C. third
   D. all of the above

24. Assessment findings in the infant exposed to varicella include all of the following EXCEPT 24.___
   A. limb atrophy
   B. angina pectoris
   C. CNS and eye abnormalities
   D. skin scars

25. The one of the following that is NOT among the available serologic tests used for the diagnosis of congenital varicella is the 25.___
   A. fluorescent antibody-to-membrane antigen (FAMA)
   B. Sabin-Feldman dye test
   C. enzyme-linked immunosorbent assay (ELISA)
   D. immune adherence hemagglutination (IAHA)

KEY (CORRECT ANSWERS)

1. C
2. D
3. D
4. B
5. D

6. A
7. D
8. C
9. D
10. C

11. D
12. B
13. D
14. A
15. C

16. D
17. C
18. D
19. D
20. D

21. A
22. C
23. A
24. B
25. B

EXAMINATION SECTION
TEST 1

DIRECTIONS: Each question or incomplete statement is followed by several suggested answers or completions. Select the one that BEST answers the question or completes the statement. *PRINT THE LETTER OF THE CORRECT ANSWER IN THE SPACE AT THE RIGHT.*

1. Which of the following CORRECTLY describe *asphyxia*? 1.____
   I. Neonatal and intrauterine asphyxia occur when there is inadequate cellular perfusion and oxygenation.
   II. The temporary cessation of respirations after an acute asphyxic episode is called primary apnea. For every 1-minute delay in artificial ventilation after an infant's last gasp in secondary apnea, the time to the first gasp is increased by approximately 2 minutes, and the time to the onset of spontaneous breathing is delayed by more than 4 minutes.
   III. Clinically, in utero asphyxia causes the fetus to have tachycardia, loss of baseline variability, late decelerations, or prolonged bradycardia. Infants born with primary apnea may have cyanosis and bradycardia, but can have good capillary filling and some muscle tone.
   IV. Infants born with secondary apnea appear bradycardic, pale, and flaccid. Spontaneous respirations may be induced by sensory stimuli.

   The CORRECT answer is:
   A. I, II B. I, III
   C. I, II, III D. I, III, IV

2. Severe fetal and neonatal asphyxia may adversely affect physiologic transitions to extrauterine life. 2.____
   After delivery, the neonate's ineffective respiratory efforts and decreased cardiac output will result in a progressive biochemical deterioration, specifically, a(n)
   I. plasma PO_2 of 0 in less than 5 minutes
   II. increase in PCO_2 of 16 mm Hg/min.
   III. decrease in pH of 0.04 units/minute
   IV. decrease in bicarbonate of 2 mEq/minute

   The CORRECT answer is:
   A. I, II, III B. I, III, IV
   C. II, III, IV D. I, II, III, IV

3. Once fetal asphyxia is diagnosed, therapeutic intervention should be coordinated between obstetric and neonatal services to allow for a timely delivery and effective coordinated resuscitation. 3.____
   The BASIC goal of resuscitation is to

A. expand the lungs and maintain adequate ventilation and oxygenation
B. maintain adequate cardiac output and tissue perfusion
C. maintain normal core temperature and avoid hypoglycemia while stabilizing the infant for transport to the nursery
D. all of the above

4. The key concept inherent in delivery room resuscitation techniques is 4.___
A. simplicity of the procedures
B. organization with a minimum of two people
C. effectiveness with continuous observation and assessment
D. anticipation and preparation

5. All of the following are conditions that may require the availability of skilled resuscitation at delivery EXCEPT 5.___
A. fetal distress
B. emergency operative delivery with general anesthesia
C. first trimester bleeding
D. breach presentation in vaginal delivery

6. The preparation for resuscitation at delivery should be done by the nursing staff by performing all of the following EXCEPT: 6.___
A. Preheating the transport incubator, making certain that the portable oxygen tanks are filled
B. Checking suction equipment for function and setting the wall vacuum regulator control at 40 to 60 mm H_2O
C. Checking availability and cleanliness of stethoscopes and pharyngoscopes
D. Checking the laryngoscope for a bright light source and appropriate blades, and checking for availability of endotracheal tubes

7. _____ is used as an emergency neonatal resuscitation drug in case of a persistent metabolic acidosis of pH less than 7.25. 7.___
A. Sodium chloride
B. Potassium chloride
C. Sodium bicarbonate
D. All of the above

8. Epinephrine is used as an emergency neonatal resuscitation drug for 8.___
A. hypotension
B. bradycardia
C. respiratory depression
D. hypoglycemia

9. In a case of severe neonatal asphyxia, all of the following are appropriate steps that should be performed EXCEPT: 9.___
A. Start immediate, vigorous resuscitation using at least three trained people working together as a swift, efficient team
B. Monitor the heart rate and other vital signs; immediately begin coordinated external cardiac massage at a rate of 100 to 120 compressions/minute

C. Place an umbilical venous catheter for required administration of drugs and volume expansion fluids and drugs
D. If the neonate has no vital signs after 10 minutes of vigorous, appropriate resuscitative interventions and drug therapy, consider discontinuing life support measures

10. Which of the following is NOT an appropriate guideline for the transport of the neonate with severe asphyxia from delivery room to nursery? 10.___
A. Transport should not interfere with ongoing care and monitoring.
B. A warmed transport incubator should be used.
C. The respiratory rate should be monitored with an electronic monitor, oximeter, or stethoscope.
D. The neonate should not be moved until adequate spontaneous or controlled ventilation is established, the heart rate is at least 100 beats/minute, and the neonate is dried and protected from excessive heat loss.

11. A known disadvantage of a self-inflating bag used as the neonatal resuscitation bag is that 11.___
A. a reservoir must be attached to deliver 100% oxygen
B. the bag cannot deliver end expiratory pressure, and it is difficult to retrofit it with an in-line manometer
C. higher pressures than the pop-off valve pressure are given with rapid ventilation
D. all of the above

12. Of the following, concerning the bag-and-mask technique used for the neonatal resuscitation, it is INCORRECT to 12.___
A. rapidly clear the mouth and pharynx of debris and fluid
B. slightly extend the head into a neutral *sniffing* position and avoid hyperextension
C. place a proper-size face mask over the neonate's nose and mouth, size 0 for infants over 2000 g and size 1 for infants under 2000 g
D. maintain a tight seal between the face and mask using the thumb, index finger, and fleshy portion of the palm between the thumb and index finger, and place the remaining fingers at the angle of and along the length of the mandible

13. Of the following, the APPROPRIATE endotracheal intubation technique for the neonatal acute resuscitation is: 13.___
A. The ET tube should lay above the carina. Using a No. 0 or No. 1 straight blade, insert the laryngoscope blade into the right corner of the neonate's mouth.

B. Nasotracheal intubation is recommended over orotracheal intubation because it can be performed rapidly without stylets and forceps.
C. Position the tip of the laryngoscope blade above the vallecula or the epiglottis.
D. Evaluate the ET tube position by auscultation for bilaterally equal cardiac sounds.

14. An ABSOLUTE indicator of the neonate's being in shock in the delivery room is 14.___
A. poor peripheral perfusion, pallor, and decreased capillary filling
B. hypotension
C. bradycardia
D. none of the above

15. _____ MUST be maintained for the management and prevention of neonatal shock. 15.___
A. Cardiac output
B. Blood pressure
C. Adequate circulating volume
D. All of the above

16. External cardiac compression to the neonate in shock is required when the heart rate is less than or equal to 16.___
A. 60 beats/minute or less than 80 beats/minute with at least 30 seconds of supported effective ventilation provided
B. 50 beats/minute or less than 70 beats/minute with at least 30 seconds of supported effective ventilation provided
C. 40 beats per minute
D. 30 beats per minute

17. The resuscitation team needs to be very careful while performing external cardiac compression on the neonate in shock, since excessive vigorous compressions can result in all of the following EXCEPT 17.___
A. pulmonary laceration
B. fractured xyphoid process
C. liver or spleen laceration
D. myocardial damage

18. The peripheral pulse used to indicate adequacy of external cardiac compressions for the neonate in shock is 18.___
A. femoral
B. brachial
C. umbilical
D. all of the above

19. All of the following are intrauterine causes of neonatal shock EXCEPT 19.___
A. hypovolemia
B. hephyxia neonatorum
C. hydrops fetalis; sepsis
D. hypoxic-induced hepatic dysfunction

20. Which of the following is NOT an extrauterine cause of neonatal shock? 20.____
   A. Delayed institution of resuscitation
   B. Respiratory distress syndrome; hyperplastic lungs
   C. Intraventricular hemorrhage; subdural hematoma
   D. Hypothermia; hypoglycemia

21. All of the following are common delivery room complications that require specialized resuscitation techniques EXCEPT 21.____
   A. meconium-stained amniotic fluid
   B. thoracic hernia
   C. bilateral choanal atresia
   D. tension pneumothorax

22. Of the following, the INCORRECT physiologic assessment finding for the normal term neonate is: 22.____
   A. The neonate's temperature drops rapidly after delivery and may not begin to stabilize for several hours unless appropriate intervention is made
   B. A normal respiratory rate is 30 to 60 breaths/minute without grunting, flaring, or retracting. A normal pulse rate is 120 to 160 beats/minute.
   C. The second period of reactivity begins between 8 and 10 hours of age. The neonate frequently has significant mucoid secretions.
   D. A full-term neonate who has not been subjected to medications or stress during labor and delivery will be awake and alert immediately after delivery

23. All of the following are appropriate laboratory data to evaluate neonatal metabolic derangements associated with thermal instability EXCEPT 23.____
   A. arterial blood gas to assess for hypoxemia and metabolic acidosis
   B. complete blood count to assess for sepsis
   C. blood galactose level to assess for hypoglycemia
   D. electrolytes to assess for hyperkalemia; BUN; serum and urine osmolality to assess hydration

24. The MOST common cause of hyperthermia in the neonatal intensive care nurseries is 24.____
   A. direct sunlight B. heaters
   C. lights D. iatrogenic

25. The normal hematocrit and hemoglobin ranges in more than 90% of term neonates are hematocrit _____% and hemoglobin _____ g/dl. 25.____
   A. 38 to 50; 12 to 16 B. 48 to 60; 16 to 20
   C. 58 to 70; 20 to 24 D. 68 to 80; 24 to 28

KEY (CORRECT ANSWERS)

1. C
2. B
3. D
4. D
5. C

6. C
7. C
8. B
9. D
10. C

11. D
12. C
13. A
14. D
15. D

16. A
17. A
18. D
19. D
20. B

21. B
22. C
23. C
24. D
25. B

TEST 2

DIRECTIONS: Each question or incomplete statement is followed by several suggested answers or completions. Select the one that BEST answers the question or completes the statement. *PRINT THE LETTER OF THE CORRECT ANSWER IN THE SPACE AT THE RIGHT.*

1. The assessment findings of the neonate with an immune anemia of RH incompatibility nature may include all of the following EXCEPT 1.____
   A. rapidly rising indirect bilirubin concentration
   B. hepatosplenomegaly
   C. decreased reticulocyte count
   D. increased nucleated red blood cells

2. If amniocentesis indicates severe anemia of RH incompatibility type or increasing bilirubin concentration in the neonate at a subsequent testing, the recommended action to take is 2.____
   A. maternal transfusion of iron
   B. intrauterine transfusion of red blood cells to the mother
   C. induction of labor
   D. all of the above

3. For severely anemic neonates with a hemoglobin concentration of less than 12 g/dl, edema or hepatosplenomegaly, an exchange transfusion should be performed immediately. This transfusion should be a 3.____
   A. transfusion with 40 ml/dg of packed red cells
   B. partial exchange transfusion with 20 ml/kg of red cells followed by a full exchange transfusion
   C. partial exchange transfusion with 40 ml/kg of packed red cells followed by a full exchange transfusion when the neonate is stable
   D. transfusion with 30 ml/kg of packed red cells

4. A positive direct Coombs' test in ABO hemolytic disease suggests severe 4.____
   A. RH incompatibility
   B. thalassemia
   C. red blood cell membrane defect
   D. hemolysis

5. Which of the following conditions is NOT required to be met to diagnose ABO hemolytic disease? 5.____
   A. Decreased number of spherocytes and microspherocytes are present in the peripheral blood of the neonate.
   B. Mild anemia, reticulocytosis, and nucleated red cells are found in the peripheral smear.

C. The mother's serum contains relatively high levels of anti-A or anti-B antibodies of IgG type.
D. Indirect hyperbilirubinemia is seen in the first 24 hours of life.

6. Both trait and homozygous states of beta thalassemia become apparent only after the infant is of age 6.___
A. 7 to 14 days B. 14 to 30 days
C. 1 to 2 months D. 2 to 3 months

7. _____ levels should be measured in newborn blood if the defects in the glycolytic pathway and pentose-phosphate shunt present as a hemolytic anemia with jaundice in the neonatal period. 7.___
A. Pyruvate kinase
B. Red blood cell enzyme
C. Glucose-6-phosphate dehydrogenase
D. All of the above

8. Diamond-Blackfan anemia, a pure red cell aplasia, is an isolated anemia caused by failure of production of _____ cells. 8.___
A. erythropoietin B. myeloid
C. erythroid D. megaloblast

9. Administering RhoGAM to an RH-negative woman within _____ hours of delivery of an RH-positive infant or fetus (if an abortion) prevents most cases of erythroblastosis fetalis. 9.___
A. 24 B. 48 C. 72 D. 96

10. The neonate with chronic blood loss may demonstrate all of the following EXCEPT 10.___
A. pallor
B. congestive heart failure
C. increased central venous pressure
D. increased central arterial pressure

11. All infants should have a central hematocrit determination performed after admittance to the neonatal intensive care unit. 11.___
If anemia is confirmed, initial laboratory examination should include all of the following EXCEPT
A. CBC; white blood cell indexes
B. reticulocyte count; direct and indirect Coombs' tests
C. determination of blood type
D. examination of the peripheral blood smear

12. If the cause of hemolysis in the neonate is not evident, the test performed to look for unstable hemoglobins, obtain red blood cell enzyme measurements to eliminate red blood cell enzyme deficiencies, and determine STORCH titers to rule out congenital infection is the _____ test. 12.___
A. Betke Kleihauer B. Heinz body
C. Direct Coombs' D. Cooley's

13. Usually hemoglobin is less than _____ g/dl. before signs and symptoms of anemia are present in the newborn. 13.___
A. 8 B. 10 C. 12 D. 14

14. An acute blood loss of _____% of the blood volume is sufficient to produce shock in the neonate which may not be reflected in the hemoglobin concentration immediately at birth. 14.___
A. 20 B. 30 C. 40 D. 50

15. If acute blood loss is suspected and the neonate is pale and limp at birth, blood pressure should be obtained and monitored, oxygen should be administered, and intravenous fluids should be started at _____ ml/kg. 15.___
A. 10 B. 20 C. 30 D. 40

16. If the neonate is anemic with signs of hypoxemia or has underlying pulmonary or cardiac disease, transfusion of red blood cells of _____ ml/kg over _____ hours can be given to increase oxygen-carrying capacity. 16.___
A. 10; 2 to 3
B. 20; 3 to 4
C. 30; 4 to 5
D. 40; 5 to 6

17. For neonates with continuing hemorrhage requiring massive blood transfusion, fresh whole blood should be used to prevent _____ that could result from transfusion with stored blood. 17.___
A. severe allergic reaction
B. infection
C. shock
D. coagulopathy

18. Using whole blood for transfusion, rather than packed cells with fresh frozen plasma, exposes the neonate to only one donor, thus decreasing the chance of _____ transmission. 18.___
A. bacterial
B. viral
C. fungal
D. all of the above

19. To be appropriate for neonatal transfusion, blood should be warmed and administered through a blood filter of at least _____ um. 19.___
A. 30 B. 40 C. 50 D. 60

20. During the neonatal blood transfusion, the nurse should know that the blood should not hang for more than _____ hours. 20.___
A. 1 to 3 B. 2 to 4 C. 3 to 5 D. 4 to 6

21. The needle size which is MOST appropriate to administer fresh blood to the neonate without significant hemolysis is _____-gauge. 21.___
A. 20 B. 22 C. 25 D. 30

22. In the delivery room, if an infant with known RH hemolytic disease is already edematous, pale, or in shock, or the cord hemoglobin is less than 12 g/dl, an immediate partial exchange transfusion with _____ ml/kg of packed red blood cells should be performed. 22.___
A. 25 B. 40 C. 55 D. 70

23. In the absence of acute symptoms, infants who are mildly anemic at birth or anemic as a result of chronic blood loss should be treated with what dosage of ferrous sulfate? 23.___
_____ mg of elemental iron/kg per _____ for _____ months.
A. 2; 8 hour; 3 B. 10; day; 4
C. 6; 8 hour; 5 D. 20; day; 6

24. Hemorrhagic disease of the newborn is USUALLY preventable by the prophylactic parenteral administration of _____ mg of vitamin K to the newborn in the first hour of life. 24.___
A. 0.5 to 1 B. 1.5 to 2 C. 2.5 to 3 D. 3.5 to 4

25. A platelet count below _____/mm^3 is ALWAYS abnormal in an infant and should be investigated. 25.___
A. 250,000 B. 200,000 C. 150,000 D. 100,000

KEY (CORRECT ANSWERS)

1. C
2. C
3. C
4. D
5. A

6. D
7. D
8. C
9. C
10. D

11. A
12. B
13. C
14. A
15. B

16. A
17. D
18. B
19. B
20. D

21. C
22. B
23. A
24. A
25. C

TEST 3

DIRECTIONS: Each question or incomplete statement is followed by several suggested answers or completions. Select the one that BEST answers the question or completes the statement. *PRINT THE LETTER OF THE CORRECT ANSWER IN THE SPACE AT THE RIGHT.*

1. A CORRECT laboratory finding for infants severely affected with disseminated intravascular coagulopathy (DIC) is a markedly 1.____
   A. reduced platelet count
   B. prolonged partial thromboplastin time (PTT)
   C. prolonged prothrombin time (PT)
   D. all of the above

2. Infants affected with passively acquired idiopathic thrombocytopenic purpura (ITP) appear healthy except for generalized petechiae. The platelet count may be less than 10,000/mm^3. 2.____
   If the infant shows increasing petechiae or other bleeding, treatment with which of the following is recommended?
   A. High-dose IV immune gamma globulin (IVIG)
   B. Low-dose IV immune alpha globulin (IVAG)
   C. High-dose IV immune beta globulin (IVBG)
   D. None of the above

3. Hemophilia A can be diagnosed at 20 weeks' gestation by measuring Factor ______ in fetal blood obtained by cordocentesis. 3.____
   A. V B. VIII C. IX D. X

4. If a newborn is bleeding, all of the following questions are useful and correct historical data that should be collected EXCEPT: 4.____
   If
   A. hemorrhagic disease of the newborn is suspected, was vitamin K given to the mother before delivery
   B. hemophilia is suspected, is there a family history of bleeding
   C. DIC is suspected, were there any obstetric complications in the delivery
   D. thrombocytopenia or platelet disorder is suspected, is there a previous history of bleeding in the mother because of ITP or SLE

5. The newborn with a bleeding problem who looks well and does not appear ill does NOT suggest which of the following causes of bleeding? 5.____
   A. Platelet defect
   B. Sepsis
   C. Vitamin K deficiency
   D. Hemophilia or other hereditary factor deficiency

6. The newborn with a bleeding problem who appears ill suggests all of the following as causes of bleeding EXCEPT 6.___
   A. DIC
   B. sepsis
   C. congenital fungal infection
   D. acute bacterial infection

7. An unusual physical finding associated with neonatal bleeding disorders is 7.___
   A. absent radii in the TAR syndrome
   B. giant hemangioma
   C. microcephaly, congenital heart disease, and chorioretinitis in congenital infection
   D. all of the above

8. The laboratory data that should be obtained in ALL infants suspected of a bleeding diathesis includes 8.___
   A. PT and PTT   B. platelet count
   C. fibrinogen   D. all of the above

9. All of the following abnormalities in screening tests are often found in bleeding newborns EXCEPT: 9.___
   If the PT
   A. is normal, the PTT is abnormally prolonged, and the platelet count is normal, suspect hemophilia B and deficiency in Factor IX
   B. and PTT are prolonged, and the platelet count is normal, suspect vitamin K deficiency as the most likely cause if the infant is well, or liver disease if the infant is ill
   C. and PTT are prolonged and the platelet count is low, suspect DIC
   D. and PTT are normal and the platelet count is low, suspect immune thrombocytopenia if the infant appears well, and renal vein thrombosis, necrotizing enterocolitis, or DIC if the infant is ill

10. If bleeding in the hemorrhagic disease of the newborn is severe or if the infant does not respond to vitamin K_1, administer _____ ml/kg fresh frozen plasma IV. 10.___
    A. 2.5   B. 5   C. 7.5   D. 10

11. _____ concentrate avoids all risk of viral infection and is the ideal product for treating hemophilia A once it is licensed. 11.___
    A. Factor V   B. Recombinant Factor VIII
    C. Factor IX   D. Recombinant Factor XI

12. Cryoprecipitate in what value can be used if Factor VIII concentrate is not available for treating neonatal hemophilia A? 12.___
    _____ pack(s) per _____ kg body weight.
    A. 1; 3   B. 2; 4   C. 3; 5   D. 4; 6

13. One cryoprecipitate pack equals _____ units of Factor VIII. 13.___
A. 50 B. 100 C. 150 D. 200

14. Neonatal bleeding resulting from severe von Willebrand's disease is extremely unusual. 14.___
If necessary, it is treated with
A. Factor V concentrate
B. Factor IX concentrate
C. Fresh frozen plasma at 20 ml/kg body weight IV
D. Cryoprecipitate 1 pack/3 kg body weight

15. If a neonate with hemophilia B is bleeding, transfuse with 15.___
A. Factor IX concentrate, 30 to 90 units/kg body weight
B. Factor XI concentrate, 50 to 80 units/kg body weight
C. fresh frozen plasma at 10 ml/kg body weight IV
D. cryoprecipitate 1 pack/3 kg body weight

16. If a neonate with afibrinogenemia is bleeding, treat with 16.___
A. 1 pack cryoprecipitate/3 kg body weight
B. fresh frozen plasma at 10 ml/kg body weight
C. 1/3 pack cryoprecipitate/kg body weight
D. all of the above

17. In the event that a neonate has any unknown hereditary coagulation factor deficiency other than hemophilia A, hemophilia B, afibrinogenemia, or von Willebrand's disease, it can be treated with 17.___
A. fresh frozen plasma at 10 ml/kg body weight IV
B. cryoprecipitate, 50 units/kg body weight
C. Factor X concentrate
D. Factor XIII concentrate

18. In disseminated intravascular coagulopathy, if the triggering event is relieved and the baby has severe DIC, treat with 18.___
A. platelet transfusions, 1 unit/kg body weight
B. fresh frozen plasma, 10 ml/kg body weight
C. fresh whole blood
D. both A and B above

19. An exchange transfusion with _____ is a reasonable method of attempting to manage DIC in neonates not responding to replacement of platelets and clotting factors. 19.___
A. fresh frozen plasma B. cryoprecipitate
C. fresh whole blood D. all of the above

20. If the triggering event persists and the baby has severe DIC, exchange transfusion is performed and heparinization is considered if the infant is septic. 20.___
Heparinization is accomplished by giving the infant 100 units of heparin per kg loading dose IV followed by continuous infusion at the rate of _____ units/kg/hour.
A. 5 to 15 B. 10 to 20 C. 15 to 25 D. 20 to 30

21. Isoimmune thrombocytopenia has an 80% chance of recurrence in subsequent pregnancies. A sample of fetal blood for platelet count can be used to decide the need for a cesarean section. 21.___
A platelet count above _____/mm^3 may allow for a safe vaginal delivery.
A. 10,000 B. 30,000 C. 50,000 D. 70,000

22. In an infant with hyperviscosity because of polycythemia, conditions associated with an increased risk of placental insufficiency include a maternal history of all of the following EXCEPT 22.___
A. preeclampsia
B. smoking
C. hypotension
D. evidence of maternal-fetal bleeding

23. Polycythemia and hyperviscosity in the neonate cause a variety of signs and symptoms involving the cardiac, respiratory, and neurologic systems. 23.___
Common clinical manifestations of these conditions do NOT include
A. plethora with peripheral cyanosis or, occasionally, pallor
B. respiratory distress that results from diminished pulmonary compliance as a result of an engorged vasculature stiffening the lungs
C. cardiomegaly, congestive heart failure
D. metabolic derangements, such as hyperglycemia and hypobilirubinemia

24. The method that most medical personnel recommend for evaluating a newborn suspected of hyperviscosity is to obtain a hematocrit 24.___
A. within the first hour after delivery; a warmed hand helps decrease falsely high values
B. when the infant is 1 to 3 hours of age
C. when the infant is 2 to 4 hours of age
D. when the infant is 4 to 6 hours of age; a warmed hand helps decrease falsely high values

25. Once it has been decided to perform a partial exchange transfusion for treating asymptomatic neonatal polycythemia, blood should be removed in _____ ml increments from the umbilical vein, and an equal amount of plasmanate should be reinfused into _____ vein. 25.___
A. 1 to 5; the radial
B. 3 to 6; the umbilical
C. 4 to 8; the peripheral
D. 5 to 10; either the umbilical or a peripheral

KEY (CORRECT ANSWERS)

1. D
2. A
3. B
4. A
5. B

6. C
7. D
8. D
9. A
10. D

11. B
12. A
13. B
14. D
15. A

16. D
17. A
18. D
19. C
20. C

21. B
22. C
23. D
24. D
25. D

EXAMINATION SECTION
TEST 1

DIRECTIONS: Each question or incomplete statement is followed by several suggested answers or completions. Select the one that BEST answers the question or completes the statement. *PRINT THE LETTER OF THE CORRECT ANSWER IN THE SPACE AT THE RIGHT.*

1. The neonate's failure to pass meconium within 48 hours after birth may indicate the congenital disorder characterized by incomplete bowel innervation and called 1.____
   A. celiac disease B. Whipple's disease
   C. Hirschprung's disease D. diverticulitis

2. All of the following are maternal prenatal sociodemographic risk factors frequently elicited from high-risk pregnancies EXCEPT 2.____
   A. low socioeconomic status; low educational level
   B. ethnic minority; emotional instability
   C. alcohol and drug abuse
   D. age under 15 or over 45

3. Which of the following is NOT a maternal risk factor concerning prenatal medical and/or obstetric disorders frequently elicited from high-risk pregnancies? 3.____
   A. Moderate to severe renal disease
   B. Moderate to severe toxemia; chronic hypertension
   C. Prior erythroblastosis fetalis; previous postmature infant
   D. Previous neonatal death; previous stillbirth

4. All of the following are maternal risk factors concerning prenatal medical and/or obstetric disorders frequently elicited from high-risk pregnancies EXCEPT 4.____
   A. prior RH sensitization; previous cesarean section
   B. habitual abortion; history of tuberculosis (TB) or PPD+
   C. history of genital herpes
   D. sickle cell disease; prior birth more than 12 lbs.

5. Prenatal physical examination findings related to maternal risk factors frequently elicited from high-risk pregnancies do NOT include 5.____
   A. acute pyelonephritis; diabetes mellitus
   B. uterine malformation; incompetent cervix
   C. polyhydramnios; oligohydramnios
   D. abnormal fetal position; hyperplasia

6. All of the following are physical examination findings related to maternal prenatal risk factors frequently elicited from high-risk pregnancies EXCEPT 6.____
   A. cervical cytology showing herpes
   B. multiple pregnancy
   C. negative serology
   D. vaginal bleeding

7. _____ are NOT considered a risk factor related to intrapartum maternal complications frequently elicited from high-risk pregnancies. 7.___
   A. Amnionitis and uterine rupture
   B. Premature rupture of membranes and premature labor
   C. Prolonged latent phase of labor and uterine tetany
   D. Precipitous labor of less than 3 hours; second stage of labor more than 2½ hours; and labor lasting over 12 hours

8. Maternal risk factors related to intrapartum complications of the placenta frequently elicited from hish-risk pregnancies include all of the following EXCEPT 8.___
   A. placenta previa
   B. postdates of more than 40 weeks' gestation
   C. meconium-stained amniotic fluid
   D. abruptio placentae

9. The one of the following which is NOT a maternal risk factor related to intrapartum fetal disorders frequently elicited from high-risk pregnancies is 9.___
   A. multiple pregnancy and fetal bradycardia
   B. fetal acidosis less than 7.25 and fetal weight less than 2000 gm.
   C. operative/vacuum delivery and difficult forceps delivery
   D. prolapsed cord and fetal tachycardia

10. All of the following maternal conditions require specialized perinatal care related to obstetric complications EXCEPT 10.___
   A. premature cervical dilation and first trimester bleeding
   B. severe preeclampsia or hypertension and multiple gestation
   C. intrauterine growth retardation with evidence of fetal distress and RH isoimmunization
   D. premature rupture of the fetal membranes and premature onset of labor

11. Which of the following is NOT considered a maternal condition requiring specialized perinatal care related to medical complications? 11.___
   A. Maternal infection that may affect the fetus or lead to premature birth
   B. Thyrotoxicosis and drug overdose
   C. Severe organic heart disease, class 2
   D. Renal disease with deteriorating function or hypertension

12. Concerning maternal conditions requiring specialized perinatal care related to surgical complications, of the following, _____ requires intensive care. 12.___
    A. trauma
    B. acute abdominal emergency
    C. thoracic emergency
    D. all of the above

13. Information regarding the tertiary center should be left with the parents. 13.___
This should include all of the following EXCEPT the
    A. location of parking facilities, nearby lodging, and rules regarding adolescents
    B. names of individuals likely to be involved with the patient's case and their telephone numbers
    C. information on the special care unit, i.e., what it is, what it does, and any particular rules or regulations regarding the special care unit
    D. exact location of the unit - address and map, plus visiting hours and hospital rules

14. The _____ is NOT a piece of neonatal transport equipment. 14.___
    A. transport incubator
    B. thermometer with skin probe
    C. IV infusion pump
    D. BP oximeter

15. Neonatal transport equipment includes all of the following supplies EXCEPT 15.___
    A. suction catheters and umbilical artery catheters
    B. intracaths, 22-24 gauge and IM pump tubing
    C. blunt needle catheter adapter and scalp vein needles
    D. thoracostomy tubes and three-way stopcocks

16. The neonatal transport equipment does NOT include the 16.___
    A. umbilical ligature and culture bottles
    B. IV filters and bacteriostatic saline
    C. Y-connectors and blood pressure monitor
    D. endotracheal tubes and Heimlich valves

17. All of the following drugs are part of neonatal transport equipment EXCEPT 17.___
    A. atropine multidose vial and albumin 10%
    B. $D_{10}W$ and D_5W, 250 ml IV bags and digoxin, 0.5 mg ampule
    C. heparin, 1000 u/ml and tolazoline, 25 mg/ml
    D. lasix, 20 mg ampule and lidocaine multidose vial

18. Which of the following drugs is NOT part of the neonatal transport equipment? 18.___
    A. Sodium bicarbonate, 0.5 mEq/ml
    B. Phenobarbital, 120 mg vial
    C. Ringer's lactate, 50 ml
    D. Prostaglandin, 500 ug/ml

19. The patient's condition and the potential limitations of each vehicle used for transport must be considered in selecting the mode of transport. 19.___
In general, for transports
  A. of less than 100 miles, a ground ambulance is the most efficient vehicle
  B. in large metropolitan areas of 100 to 250 miles, a helicopter is the better choice
  C. beyond 250 miles, fixed-wing aircrafts have a distinct advantage
  D. all of the above

20. The maternal transport equipment related to regionalization and transport in perinatal care includes all of the following groups EXCEPT 20.___
  A. IV infusion pump and IV stand/poles
  B. blood pressure monitor and fetal heart rate monitor
  C. stainless steel buckets and basins and scissors
  D. speculum and suction apparatus

21. Of the following supplies, the group that is NOT part of the maternal transport equipment used for the regionalization and transport in perinatal care is 21.___
  A. Kelly clamps, 4, suture set, and assorted suture material
  B. pudental block set and D5W, 1000 ml
  C. Ringer's lactate, 250 ml, and blood administration set
  D. assorted angiocaths and suction bulb

22. In relation to regionalization and transport in perinatal care, which of the following is NOT an appropriate drug used and required in maternal transport equipment? 22.___
  A. Narcan, adult, 0.4 mg ampule; pitocin, 10 u/ml
  B. Terbutaline, 80 mg in 500 ml D5 $\frac{1}{4}$NS; lasix, 120 mg
  C. Lidocaine, 1%, without epinephrine; methergine, 0.2 mg/ml
  D. Ritodrine, 150 mg/500 ml; demerol, 50 and 75 mg ampules

23. Assuming adequate placental function and perfusion, elevations in maternal glucose lead to fetal hyperglycemia and increased fetal insulin production. 23.___
Repeated or continued elevations in blood glucose result in
  A. fetal hyperinsulinism
  B. alterations in the utilization of glucose and other nutrients
  C. altered patterns of growth and development
  D. all of the above

24. The various complications of maternal diabetes are also associated with fetal and neonatal problems, including all of the following EXCEPT 24.____
A. growth retardation
B. chronic hypoxia
C. postmaturity
D. intrauterine demise

25. In terms of predicting perinatal morbidity and mortality, the *prognostically bad signs of pregnancy*, first identified by Pedersen in the 1960's, are especially significant and continue to be useful predictors of increased fetal and neonatal risk. 25.____
Of the following, only _____ is NOT among these signs.
A. diabetic ketoalkalosis
B. pregnancy-induced hypertension
C. pyelonephritis
D. maternal noncompliance

26. In preparing for the delivery of an infant of a diabetic (IDM), along with indicators of fetal growth and well-being, the neonatal team should consider all of the following EXCEPT the 26.____
A. classification of maternal diabetes
B. quality of metabolic control throughout the pregnancy and labor
C. fetal complications
D. duration of the pregnancy

27. In rare cases, the offspring of women with Grave's disease may themselves be afflicted with this condition. In the fetus and neonate, the one of the following that does NOT show evidence of this condition is 27.____
A. decreased heart rate
B. growth retardation
C. goiter
D. congestive heart failure

28. Phenylketonuria (PKU) is a genetic disorder in which an enzymatic defect precludes the conversion of the essential amino acid 28.____
A. phenylalanine to cystine
B. tyrosine to phenylalanine
C. phenylalanine to lysine
D. phenylalanine to tyrosine

29. The metabolic derangement in phenylketonuria (PKU) is evidenced by the excessive accumulation of phenylalanine in the maternal 29.____
A. urine
B. spinal fluid
C. lymphatic drainage
D. blood

30. Several studies about PKU have identified improved long-term outcomes when desirable phenylalanine levels of less than _____ mg/dl are achieved before or early in pregnancy and maintained throughout. 30.____
A. 2 to 8
B. 8 to 14
C. 14 to 20
D. 20 to 26

KEY (CORRECT ANSWERS)

1. C	11. C	21. C
2. D	12. D	22. B
3. C	13. A	23. D
4. D	14. D	24. C
5. D	15. B	25. A
6. C	16. C	26. C
7. D	17. A	27. A
8. B	18. C	28. D
9. B	19. D	29. D
10. A	20. D	30. A

TEST 2

DIRECTIONS: Each question or incomplete statement is followed by several suggested answers or completions. Select the one that BEST answers the question or completes the statement. *PRINT THE LETTER OF THE CORRECT ANSWER IN THE SPACE AT THE RIGHT.*

1. Regardless of the underlying etiology, pregnancy outcome relates MOST closely to 1.____
   A. hypotension and renal glucosuria
   B. hypertension and hepatic insufficiency
   C. hypotension and hepatic cholecystitis
   D. hypertension and renal insufficiency

2. Under which of the following circumstances would women rarely become pregnant, but if pregnancy does occur, it would be associated with significant perinatal morbidity and mortality? 2.____
   A. Hemofiltration
   B. Renal transplantation
   C. Dialysis
   D. Hepatic insufficiency

3. Infants born after maternal renal transplantation are commonly called 3.____
   A. preterm
   B. term
   C. postterm
   D. all of the above

4. _____ is a potent teratogen that is contraindicated in pregnancy and is associated with spontaneous abortion, craniofacial anomalies, intrauterine growth retardation, hypoplasia of the fingers and nails, congenital heart defects, and mental retardation. 4.____
   A. Aminopterin
   B. Trimethadione
   C. Actinomycin D
   D. Vincristine

5. Infants born to mothers treated with anticonvulsants, especially barbiturates, may exhibit which of the following signs of generalized depression? 5.____
   A. Decreased respiratory effort
   B. Poor muscle tone
   C. Feeding difficulties
   D. All of the above

6. There have been reports of abnormal clotting and hemorrhage in the offspring of women treated with 6.____
   A. phenytoin
   B. phenobarbital
   C. primidone
   D. all of the above

7. Myasthenia gravis is an autoimmune disorder in which a dearth of acetylcholine receptor (AChR) results in _____ dysfunction. 7.____
   A. neuromuscular
   B. musculoskeletal
   C. renal
   D. neuroskeletal

8. Affected infants born to mothers with myasthenia gravis usually present at birth, or within the first 24 hours of life, with 8.____
   A. generalized weakness
   B. diminished suck and swallow
   C. decreased respiratory effort that may require mechanical support
   D. all of the above

9. The neonatal manifestations of systemic lupus erythematosus (SLE) are attributed to the placental transfer of maternal antibodies to the fetus. 9.____
   Findings in the neonate do NOT include
   A. transient lupus-like rash
   B. thrombocytopenia
   C. renal abnormalities
   D. cardiac abnormalities

10. A strong association has been established between maternal antiRo (SS-A) antibodies and congenital heart block in the offspring of women with SLE. 10.____
   The heart block is often identified prenatally and infants are treated, after delivery, with
   A. corticosteroids
   B. acetylsalicylic acid
   C. antibiotics
   D. cardiac pacemakers

11. Significant reductions in maternal cardiac output create decreased uterine blood flow and diminished placental perfusion with a resulting impairment in the exchange of nutrients, oxygen, and metabolic wastes. 11.____
   Possible fetal and neonatal consequences include all of the following EXCEPT
   A. spontaneous abortion
   B. intrauterine growth retardation
   C. peripheral nervous system damage
   D. neonatal asphyxia and intrauterine demise

12. Oral anticoagulants, specifically warferin (coumarin), have been associated with fetal malformations, including nasal hypoplasia and epiphyseal stippling when administered to the mother during the _____ trimester. 12.____
   A. first
   B. second
   C. third
   D. all of the above

13. The incidence of warfarin embyopathy is estimated at _____%; an additional _____% of these pregnancies are complicated by perinatal hemorrhage with associated risk of fetal death, prematurity, and neonatal hemorrhage. 13.____
   A. 5 to 15; 1 to 5
   B. 15 to 25; 5 to 10
   C. 25 to 35; 10 to 15
   D. none of the above

14. Propranolol, a beta-blocker commonly used to treat both maternal hypertension and dysrhythmias, acts as a uterine stimulant and is a possible cause of preterm labor. 14.___
It is also associated with neonatal depression, including decreased respiratory effort and bradycardia at the time of delivery, as well as all of the following complications in the newborn period EXCEPT
A. hypoglycemia
B. polycythemia
C. thrombocytopenia
D. hyperbilirubinemia

15. In general, due to its being a cause of serious damages in the neonate, diuretic use is restricted to women with 15.___
A. pulmonary edema
B. acute cardiac failure
C. acute renal failure
D. all of the above

16. Fetal risks related to uncontrolled maternal asthma include all of the following EXCEPT 16.___
A. low birth weight
B. hypocalcemia
C. prematurity
D. hypoglycemia

17. Fetal risks related to maternal cystic fibrosis, caused primarily by maternal hypoxemia and infection, do NOT include 17.___
A. prematurity
B. intrauterine growth retardation
C. neonatal hypoglycemia
D. perinatal death

18. Maternal smoking is associated with all of the following EXCEPT 18.___
A. reductions in both neonatal birth weight and length
B. placental dysfunction and increased incidence of placental abruptions and previas
C. renal insufficiency
D. intrauterine fetal demise

19. Maternal deficiencies of vitamins and minerals have NOT been linked to 19.___
A. spontaneous abortion and congestive heart failure
B. megaloblastic anemia and congenital anomalies
C. skeletal abnormalities
D. muscular atrophy

20. Vitamin overdosage in the mother, especially of fat-soluble vitamins, has been implicated in fetal abnormalities. 20.___
Vitamin A overdose has been associated with
A. kidney malformations
B. neural tube defects
C. hydrocephalus
D. all of the above

21. Maternal vitamin overdosage has been implicated in fetal abnormalities. 21.____
Vitamin D overdose has NOT been associated with ______ defects.
A. cardiac
B. musculoskeletal
C. neurologic
D. renal

22. Maternal cardiovascular support is crucial to fetal well-being. The net effect of the chronic maternal blood loss on the fetus is decreased oxygenation and impaired nutrient delivery. 22.____
The MOST common cause of hemorrhage late in pregnancy is
A. placental abruption and placenta previa
B. hypofibrinogenemia
C. metrorrhagia
D. infection

23. Preeclampsia, which has a significant effect on neonatal outcome, is a type of pregnancy-induced hypertension and is a condition in which hypertension, accompanied by proteinuria and edema, develops during the ______ of pregnancy in women with or without preexisting hypertensive disease. 23.____
A. first half
B. first trimester
C. second half
D. second trimester

24. Preeclampsia is LEAST common in 24.____
A. primigravidas
B. women 16 to 35 years of age
C. multiple gestations and molar pregnancies
D. women with a family history of this disorder

25. The fetal and neonatal risks associated with preeclampsia include all of the following EXCEPT 25.____
A. prematurity
B. intrauterine growth retardation
C. perinatal asphyxia and polycythemia
D. thrombocytopenia

26. The development of HELLP syndrome during pregnancy is an indication, regardless of the gestational age of the fetus, for 26.____
A. diabetes
B. renal disease
C. respiratory disease
D. delivery

27. A birth before ______ weeks' gestation which poses an unparalleled threat to neonatal survival and well-being is defined as a preterm labor. 27.____
A. 35
B. 37
C. 39
D. 41

28. All of the following factors related to maternal history are associated with preterm labor and delivery EXCEPT 28.____
   A. chronic disease and diabetes
   B. renal disease and cardiovascular disease
   C. underweight before pregnancy and previous preterm labor
   D. smoking and age below 15 and above 30

29. Which of the following factors related to current pregnancy is NOT associated with preterm labor and delivery? 29.____
   A. Inadequate weight gain and retained IUD
   B. Acute maternal illness and polyhydramnios
   C. Isoimmunization and postpartum hemorrhage
   D. multiple gestation and premature rupture of the membranes

30. ______ is associated with preterm labor and delivery. 30.____
   A. Intrauterine fetal demise
   B. Fetal anomalies
   C. Infection
   D. All of the above

KEY (CORRECT ANSWERS)

1. D	11. C	21. B
2. C	12. A	22. A
3. A	13. B	23. C
4. B	14. C	24. B
5. D	15. D	25. D
6. D	16. B	26. D
7. A	17. C	27. B
8. D	18. C	28. D
9. C	19. D	29. C
10. D	20. D	30. D

TEST 3

DIRECTIONS: Each question or incomplete statement is followed by several suggested answers or completions. Select the one that BEST answers the question or completes the statement. *PRINT THE LETTER OF THE CORRECT ANSWER IN THE SPACE AT THE RIGHT.*

1. Beta-sympathomimetic agents are commonly used as a means of interrupting preterm labor. 1.____
Although they are effective in prolonged gestation, they are also associated with all of the following maternal complications EXCEPT
   A. tachycardia and dysrhythmias
   B. hyperglycemia
   C. hyperkalemia
   D. anxiety, nausea, and vomiting

2. Beta-sympathomimetic agents, which are commonly used as a means of interrupting preterm labor, are effective in prolonged gestation but are also associated with fetal 2.____
   A. tachycardia and hyperglycemia
   B. bradycardia and hyperglycemia
   C. tachycardia and hypoglycemia
   D. bradycardia and hypoglycemia

3. Neonates born after maternal beta-sympathomimetic therapy may develop ______ in response to in utero hyperglycemia and overproduction of insulin. 3.____
   A. tachycardia
   B. hyperglycemia
   C. bradycardia
   D. hypoglycemia

4. Neonatal consequences of maternal magnesium administration do NOT include 4.____
   A. decreased muscle tone
   B. drowsiness
   C. decreased serum calcium levels
   D. decreased serum potassium levels

5. Maternal barbiturate administration during labor has all of the following effects on the fetus and newborn EXCEPT 5.____
   A. CNS and PNS depression
   B. respiratory depression
   C. slowed metabolism
   D. lethargy, decreased tone, and feeding difficulties

6. Fetus and neonatal effects are related to the dose, route, and timing of maternal administration of narcotics. 6.____
Which of the following is NOT an effect caused by maternal narcotics administration during labor on the fetus and newborn?

A. CNS depression
B. Decreased muscle tone and reflexes
C. Decreased respiratory effort and responsiveness
D. Fetal tachycardia

7. Maternal tranquilizer administration during labor has all of the following effects on the fetus and newborn EXCEPT 7.___
A. fetal tachycardia and decreased beat-to-beat variability
B. impaired thermoregulation
C. CNS depression
D. depressed respiratory effort and apnea

8. Related to the duration and depth of anesthesia, the administration of maternal general (inhalation) anesthesia causes _____ in the fetus and newborn. 8.___
A. CNS depression B. respiratory depression
C. decreased responsiveness D. all of the above

9. The non-stress test (NST) was formalized by requiring _____ episodes of fetal heart rate accelerations of at least 15 beats/minute within a 20 minute period, which is considered *reactive* and a sign of fetal well-being. 9.___
A. one B. two C. three D. four

10. Which of the following is NOT correct about the non-stress test (NST)? 10.___
A. This test seems to reflect the state of fetal CNS oxygenation at the time of the test.
B. Since it does not entail the production of uterine contractions, there are fewer potential problems or contraindications to the NST.
C. It evaluates uteroplacental reserve.
D. Since it is quicker and easier to conduct, the NST is often the first-line screening test of fetal well-being.

11. Congenital malformations or a specific dysmorphic syndrome in offspring has been associated with the opioid 11.___
A. heroin B. methadone
C. meperidene D. none of the above

12. Cocaine, a non-opioid substance, crosses the placenta by simple diffusion. 12.___
This occurs because it possesses
A. high lipid solubility
B. low molecular weight
C. low ionization at physiologic pH
D. all of the above

13. Cocaine has a marked vasoconstrictive property, which decreases blood flow to the placenta and fetus, contributing to _____ in the fetus. 13.___
   A. growth retardation and hypoxia
   B. fetal toxicity
   C. respiratory depression
   D. impaired thermoregulation

14. Alcohol has been shown to cause all of the following in the fetus EXCEPT 14.___
   A. disruption of protein synthesis
   B. impaired cellular growth
   C. impaired cellular differentiation and migration
   D. diminished RNS synthesis

15. Alcohol interferes with the transport of _____ across the placenta to the fetus, thus altering embryonic organization, with intrauterine growth retardation and chronic fetal hypoxia as the result. 15.___
   A. proteins B. amino acids
   C. carbohydrates D. essential vitamins

16. Neonatal abstinence is described as a generalized disorder characterized by all of the following EXCEPT 16.___
   A. CNS hyperirritability
   B. gastrointestinal dysfunction
   C. fetal neonatal toxicity
   D. vague autonomic symptoms such as yawning, sneezing, mottled color, and fever

17. The onset of drug withdrawal symptoms in narcotic abstinence syndrome (NAS) varies from minutes or hours after birth to _____ weeks of age. 17.___
   A. 2 B. 4 C. 6 D. 8

18. Most infants at birth who have been exposed to narcotics appear physically _____ and behaviorally _____. 18.___
   A. normal;abnormal B. abnormal; abnormal
   C. abnormal; normal D. normal; normal

19. One of the most serious consequences of neonatal abstinence is the development of seizures. Seizures occur in about _____ percent of heroin-exposed neonates. 19.___
   A. 1 to 2 B. 3 to 5 C. 6 to 8 D. 7 to 9

20. Seizures occur in about _____ percent of methadone-exposed neonates. 20.___
   A. 1 to 3 B. 3 to 5 C. 5 to 7 D. 7 to 9

21. Infants experiencing narcotic abstinence syndrome (NAS) frequently exhibit all of the following respiratory symptoms EXCEPT 21.___

A. excessive nasal secretion and chest retraction
B. stuffy nose and nasal flaring
C. intermittent cyanosis and apnea
D. slow respirations

22. Increased severity of the respiratory symptoms in infants experiencing narcotic abstinence syndrome (NAS) may occur when the infant 22.___
A. regurgitates
B. aspirates
C. develops aspiration pneumonia
D. all of the above

23. The abstinence scoring sheet lists a total of _____ symptoms most commonly observed in the opioid-exposed neonate and recorded as single entities or in several categories if they occur in varying degrees of severity. 23.___
A. 11 B. 21 C. 31 D. 41

24. According to the abstinence scoring test, what score is considered the point of optimal behavior and neurologic state in which the infant should be maintained? 24.___
A. 0 B. 1 to 3 C. 4 to 7 D. 8 to 10

25. A score of _____ on the abstinence scoring test is considered a point where need for pharmacologic intervention to control withdrawal symptomatology arises. 25.___
A. 17 B. 1 to 3 C. 8 to 10 D. 14 to 16

26. Which of the following statements is NOT correct about the salient points to be considered when using the Neonatal Abstinence Scoring System? 26.___
A. The first score should be recorded approximately 2 hours following admission to the nursery.
B. All infants should be scored at 4-hour intervals unless high scores indicate a need for more frequent scoring.
C. The infant is scored if prolonged crying is exhibited, even though it may not be high-pitched in quality.
D. Respirations are counted for at least 15 seconds.

27. The pharmacologic agents MOST commonly used in the treatment of drug withdrawal in the neonate include 27.___
A. agonists and digitoxin
B. paregoric and phenobarbital
C. procainamide and quinidine
D. digoxin and phenytoin

28. Complications of excessive pharmacologic treatment include all of the following EXCEPT 28.___
A. diminished or absent reflexes: Moro, sucking, swallowing, Galant, Perez, tonic neck, corneal, and grasp

B. absence of response to painful stimuli
C. hypothermia and altered respirations
D. truncal (central) or circumoral cyanosis or persistent mottling not associated with ambient temperature decreases

29. Rapid physiologic transition from intrauterine to extrauterine environments must be made at birth. Effective rhythmic respirations should be initiated within _____ seconds of delivery. 29.___
A. 5 to 10 B. 10 to 15 C. 15 to 30 D. 30 to 45

30. Which of the following statements regarding the mechanism of generation of the initial breath in the neonate is CORRECT? 30.___
A. The initial breath may generate from 20 to 70 cm. H_2O of negative intrathoracic pressure to expand the collapsed alveoli.
B. A rapid decrease in pulmonary vascular resistance occurs after lung expansion, resulting in increased pulmonary perfusion and oxygenation.
C. A rapid increase in pulmonary circulation occurs after lung expansion, resulting in increased pulmonary perfusion and oxygenation.
D. All of the above

KEY (CORRECT ANSWERS)

1. C	11. D	21. D
2. A	12. D	22. D
3. D	13. A	23. B
4. D	14. D	24. A
5. A	15. B	25. C
6. D	16. C	26. D
7. C	17. A	27. B
8. D	18. D	28. B
9. B	19. A	29. D
10. C	20. C	30. D

OBSTETRICAL NURSING CARE

Introduction

a. *General*: Obstetrics is the branch of medicine primarily concerned with the health and safety of the childbearing woman and her newborn baby. In health care programs, emphasis is placed on complete maternity care, which includes special obstetrical health supervision and management during three distinct periods: (1) prenatal, (2) labor and delivery, and (3) postpartum (after childbirth).

(1) *Prenatal care*: This includes the medical supervision and education of the expectant mother throughout her pregnancy. Her physical health is checked thoroughly on her initial visit to the doctor and is watched closely during subsequent regularly scheduled visits. Effective prenatal care is essentially preventive medical care, to reduce the possibility of complications developing either during or following pregnancy, to prepare the prospective mother and father for parenthood, and to increase the chances of giving birth to a healthy, normal baby.

NOTE: Although prenatal care starts with the initial visit of the pregnant woman to the doctor, it is important to emphasize that basic preparation for childbirth and parenthood should start long before the initial prenatal clinic visit; this phase of health care starts with the education of men (prospective fathers) and women (prospective mothers) to the responsibilities of adulthood and family living. The building of healthy attitudes toward sex, hygiene, and family living should start in early adulthood.

(2) *Childbirth*: Care in childbirth includes the assistance and management of mother and infant during and immediately following labor and delivery. Labor is the series of processes by which the fetus (unborn baby), placenta, and fetal membrane are expelled from the uterus into the outside world; delivery is the actual birth of the baby. In the normal course of events, the mother has been instructed during her prenatal period about the beginning signs of labor and about entering the hospital at that time for care and medical management. Special, segregated mother and newborn-baby care facilities are established on the obstetrics (OB) service for maternity patients. The mother and baby are separated from contact with medical-surgical patients so that the special needs of the "non-sick" mother and newborn can be met as safely as possible. Nursing personnel assigned to the OB service are usually involved in the care of obstetrical patients only, and unassigned personnel have little or no contact with the OB patient and newborn infant.

(3) *Post partum care*: This includes the immediate care of the mother following delivery and her follow-up care. The post partum period is called the puerperium, which is the 6- to 8-week period of time following childbirth during which the organs of reproduction return to normal size and function. Although the mother is discharged from the hospital usually within 3 to 4 days following delivery, she is not discharged from the maternity care program until she has had a satisfactory 6-week follow-up physical examination and interview with the doctor. This follow-up care program is a means of assuring the recovery and good health of the mother and an opportunity for the obstetrician to see

that the baby is under the care of a pediatrician (or well baby clinic) to assure his health and normal development.

b. *Role of the Medical Specialist*: The medical specialist will normally carry out any OB nursing assignment under the direct supervision of a doctor and professional nurse. Specific policies and procedures in written form are provided, covering day-to-day routine operation of ward or clinic activities and including directives for unusual circumstances. WAC medical specialists are more apt to benefit from the educational experience and training in OB clinics and wards, since it is customary to assign female nonprofessional personnel to the OB service for direct patient care duties. However, it is the male medical specialist who is most likely to be confronted with the emergency situation of a medically unattended and imminent childbirth outside the hospital setting. In his assignment as aidman in a disaster relief situation, as dispensary specialist in an area removed from a hospital, or as a hospital ambulance attendant, he may be the only one available to aid the mother and baby. He should, therefore, have some definite information on what takes place immediately before, during and after normal childbirth. With some background information, he will be able to give competent assistance at a time of crisis. The birth of a baby is a normal, natural, physical event, but it is also a deeply emotional experience for both the mother and the individual assisting her. In an emergency situation, the assistant must know how to help the mother help herself. The mother needs the reassurance that a competent medical specialist is present and can help her. The procedure for emergency childbirth discussed in this section is a guide for the medical specialist who is at the scene of imminent childbirth when circumstances make it impossible to obtain the services of a medical officer or nurse. Professional care must be sought as quickly as possible following the necessary emergency measures.

The Mother and Baby at Onset of Labor

A full-term pregnancy lasts approximately 280 days (10 lunar months) from first day of last normal menstrual period. To calculate the EDC (expected date of confinement), subtract 3 months and add 7 days from the first day of last normal menstrual period. The mother's body has been physiologically prepared for labor and delivery by changes that have taken place throughout the prenatal period. Similarly, the baby has grown and developed so that it is ready for existence in the outside world. Nature has therefore prepared both for this great event. The typical, normal relationships of the bodies of the mother and of a full-term baby are illustrated in figures 7-1 and 7-2.

a. *The Baby and the Birth Canal.* Toward the end of a full-term pregnancy, the baby has usually positioned itself head down, with the buttocks toward the fundus (fig. 7-1(a)). The head-down position, with the baby's head already descended through the broad upper inlet of the mother's pelvis, brings the uterus downward and forward. The lower part of the mother's abdomen becomes very prominent. The mother has less pressure in the upper abdomen and increased pressure in the pelvic region. The baby's position is now most favorable for passage through the cervix (fig. 7-1 (b)) to the vagina (birth canal) (fig. 7-1(c)).

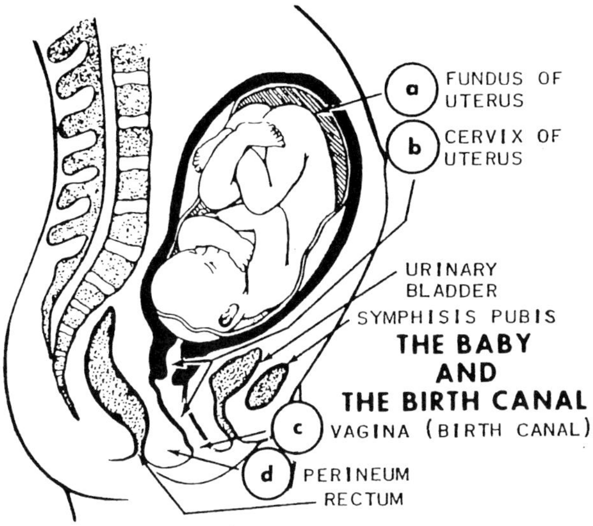

Figure 7-1. The baby and the birth canal.

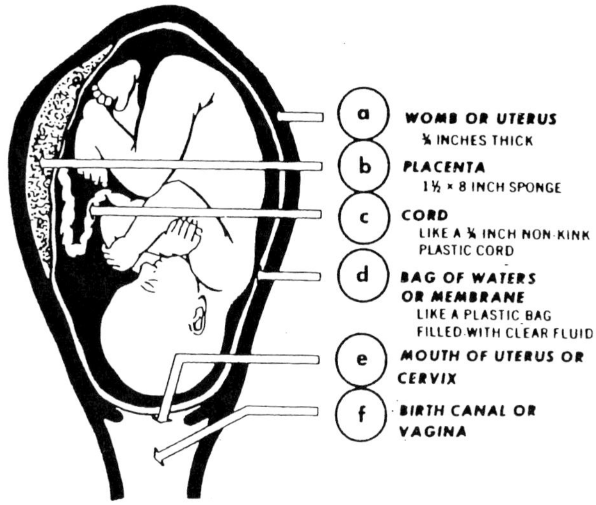

Figure 7-2. The baby and intrauterine structures.

b. *The Baby and Intrauterine Structures*

(1) *The uterus.* The wall of the uterus (fig. 7-2(a)) becomes thin and its muscle fibers stretch and hypertrophy during the expansion of the uterine cavity to accommodate the developing baby and the essential intrauterine accessory structures (placenta, fetal membranes, and umbilical cord). The special arrangement of smooth muscle and vascular tissue of the uterus allows for great expansion in pregnancy and also for forcible contractions during labor and delivery. Additionally, the arrangement of muscle fibers make it possible for the uterus to contract after delivery, to constrict blood vessels and prevent maternal hemorrhage.

(2) *The placenta.* The placenta (fig. 7-2 (b)) is the special intrauterine organ that develops during the early months of pregnancy and serves the unborn baby throughout its intrauterine life. The placenta normally is firmly attached (implanted) to the inner vascular wall at the main body of the uterus. It functions primarily as a go-between organ by which the baby receives oxygen and nutrients from the mother's blood and disposes of waste products for absorption into the mother's blood. The exchange of nutrients and wastes takes place through a special sieve-like membrane in the placenta; the baby's blood and the mother's do not mix. The placenta also produces hormones, such as estrogen and progesterone to sustain the pregnancy. At full term, the placenta is about 8 inches in diameter, about 1-1/2 inches thick, and weighs about 1 pound, varying in size and weight with the baby (it will be about one-sixth of the baby's weight). After the baby is born, the placental function is completed and the placenta separates from its attachment to the uterine wall and is delivered as the afterbirth.

(3) *Fetal membranes.* The double-walled membranous sac filled with watery fluid (bag of waters) is called the fetal membranes (fig. 7-2 (d)). The inner surface of the sac is called the amnion and the fluid in which the baby floats is amniotic fluid. The amount is variable, usually from 500 to 1000 ml. The plastic-like sac of fluid insulates and protects the baby during pregnancy; during labor, a portion of the fluid-filled sac is usually forced ahead of the baby and serves as a resilient wedge to help dilate the cervix. The membranes are attached to the margins of the placenta and the placental end of the umbilical cord.

(4) *Umbilical cord.* The umbilical cord (fig. 7-2(c)) is the unborn baby's lifeline, attaching the baby to the placenta. The cord contains three blood vessels (one vein and two arteries), in a spiral arrangement and a protective gelatinous substance called Wharton's jelly. The vein carries oxygenated blood to the fetus. The arteries carry deoxygenated blood back to the intervillous spaces in the placenta. The cord structure, plus the blood traveling through it at about 4 miles per hour, keeps the cord from kinking, which would obstruct the vital blood flow to and from the placenta. As the baby is born, the cord resembles a sturdy plastic rope; it is about 22 inches in length and about 1 inch in diameter.

Stages of Labor

For the purposes of this manual, labor is considered to progress normally in three distinct stages—

a. *First Stage (Stage of Dilation):* During this period, the cervix (fig. 7-2(e)) becomes fully dilated to allow the baby's head to come through from the body of the uterus to the birth canal (fig. 7-2(f)).

b. *Second Stage (Stage of Expulsion):* During this period, the baby moves through the birth canal and is born.

c. *Third Stage (Placental Stage):* During this period, the placenta separates from the uterine wall, and the placenta and its attached fetal membranes are expelled from the uterus.

Recognition of the Progress of Labor (First to Second Stage)

The first signs of labor may be noticeable only to the mother as she experiences a dull, low backache and cramping pains in the lower abdomen. As labor progresses, it is important for the mother and the assistant to be aware of the significance of signs, which although variable, are typical and will be noticeable to both.

a. Irregular contractions become regular, last longer and become stronger. The medical specialist should know how to time and evaluate the force of contractions by a method that is more accurate than just observing the patient's actions or facial expression, since patients react differently. A recommended method is as follows:

(1) Place your hand on the patient's abdomen, just above her umbilicus, to feel the involuntary tightening and relaxation of the uterine muscles.

(2) Time the contraction (in seconds) from the moment the uterus first tightens until it is completely relaxed. Time the interval (in minutes) from the start of one contraction to the start of the next. The intensity, whether or not the patient complains of pain, is evaluated by the sense of hardness felt during the contraction; with an intense (strong) contraction, the fingers cannot indent the abdominal surface.

(3) When contractions recur at regular 3- to 4-minute intervals, last from 50 to 60 seconds (or longer), and feel very hard, the patient is considered to be in the latter part of the first stage of labor. The cervix is probably dilating rapidly. She should not be walking about and should not be left alone—the second stage will probably begin very soon.

b. Membranes may rupture ("bag of waters broken"). In addition to increasing frequency, duration and intensity of contractions, there may be a rupture of membranes during the first stage, which would be indicated by a gush of watery fluid from the vagina. Some blood-tinged mucus ("bloody show") may appear on the patient's clothing also. As labor progresses, both will probably increase. In an emergency situation, no attempt should be made to wipe away secretions from the vagina since extreme care must be used to prevent any contamination of the birth canal. When these vaginal discharges are present, it is usually advisable to keep the patient lying down. If a clean towel is available, it can be placed under her buttocks to absorb any moisture. Check the fetal heart sounds following membrane rupture. Lack of sounds may indicate a possible cord prolapse.

c. During the first stage of labor the mother should be encouraged to relax and "let herself go" with each contraction. As each contraction starts, abdominal breathing or quiet breathing with mouth closed will help this relaxation. She will waste strength and energy by attempting to bear down or push.

d. Toward the end of the first stage of labor, there will be a noticeable increase in the strength and frequency of contractions and an increasing sense of pressure on the rectum. There is involuntary contraction of the abdominal muscles and an increasing feeling of urgency by the mother to bear down and push, as for a bowel movement. This indicates she is rapidly nearing the second or expulsion stage—the cervix is probably fully open, and the baby is beginning its passage through the birth canal (fig. 7-3). The mother will often make an involuntary deep grunting moan with each increasingly strong contraction. The medical specialist must now be prepared to assist with the imminent delivery of the baby.

Assisting With an Emergency Delivery (Second Stage of Labor)

a. *General instructions.*

(1) Be calm. Reassure the mother that you are there to help her with the delivery.

(2) Use aseptic technique to the greatest extent possible under the circumstances.

(3) Be prepared to administer first aid measures for both mother and baby. These measures include possible respiratory and cardiac resuscitation for the baby, in addition to prevention of shock and control of hemorrhage for the mother.

(4) Protect the mother to the greatest extent possible from onlookers or curious bystanders.

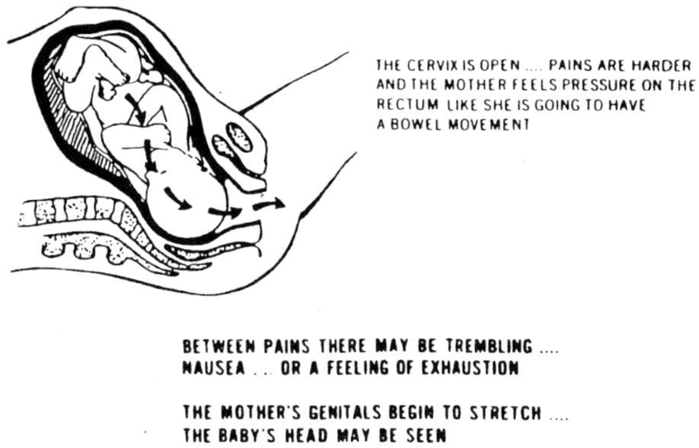

Figure 7–3. Beginning of second stage.

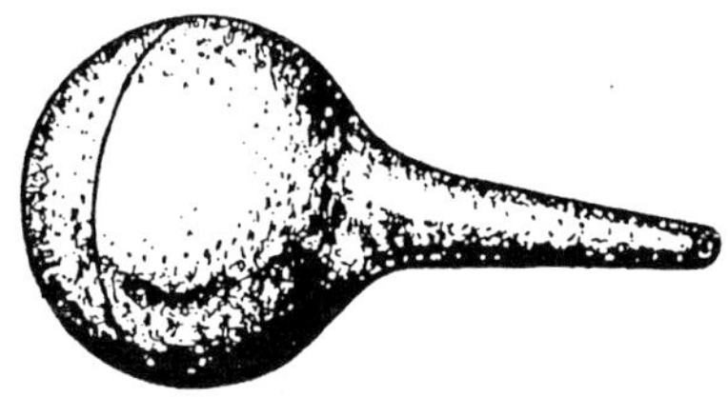

Figure 7–4. Syringe, ear and ulcer.

b. *Desirable Equipment*: A basic sterile obstetric pack should be available for use at the time of an emergency delivery in every ambulance dispatched to an emergency maternity call or in every dispensary subject to such an emergency call. This commercially prepared item is sealed in a plastic envelope. A similar pack may be prepared by a local CMS unit.

(1) The recommended equipment includes the following items:

Sterile pack, containing-
- Sheets, 3
- Towels, 4
- Pads, gauze, 4 inch x 4 inch, 12
- Sanitary pads, 2
- Syringe, rubber, 1*
- Blanket (baby receiving blanket), 1

In carton or outside of pack—
- Sterile gloves
- Germicide wipes, foil-wrapped

* The recommended syringe (fig 7-4) is called an "ear and ulcer syringe." It is used for gentle p.r.n. aspiration of secretions from the baby's mouth.

(2) If no sterile equipment is available, use the cleanest items at hand—towels or parts of the mother's clothing. If newspapers are available, place some under her. When possible, place a raincoat or blanket under her if she must lie on the ground.

c. *Preparation for the Delivery.*

(1) Assist the patient to lie on her back with knees bent and separated as far apart as possible.

(2) Remove any constricting clothing or push it above her waist.

(3) Have the best possible light directed toward her genital area. Observe for gapping of the vagina and bulging of the perineum (fig. 7-1(d)). With each contraction, the baby's head may be visible (fig. 7-5 (a)) as the labia opens wider.

(4) If equipment is available—

(a) Cleanse your hands with germicide wipes.

(b) Place pack convenient to use. Open pack.

(c) Remove one sheet, touching only the corners.

(d) Between contractions, when the mother can concentrate on what you are telling her to do, ask her to raise her hips. Place one fold of the sheet well under her hips and unfold it toward her feet.

(e) If time permits, use a second sheet to cover lower abdomen and legs, leaving perineal area uncovered. (Apply in diamond shape, turning back fourth corner, as in figure 5-32).

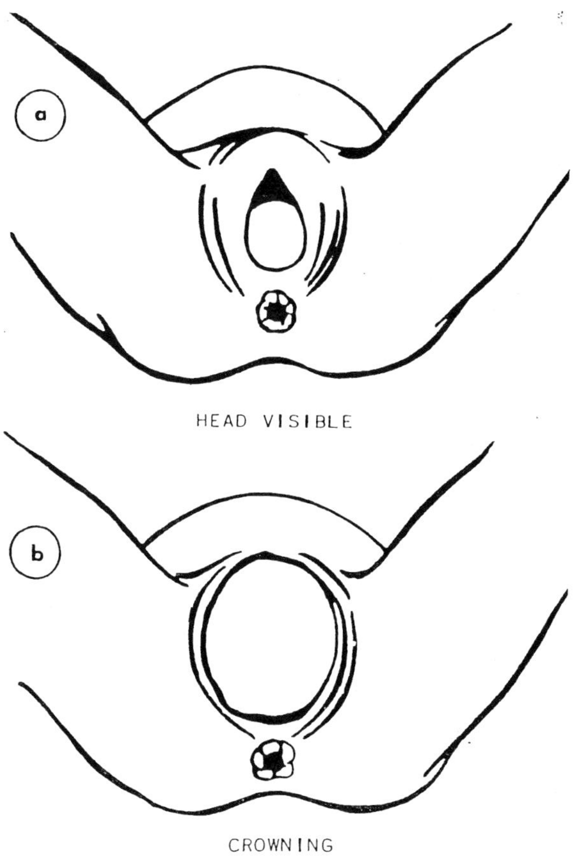

Figure 7–5. Second stage: crowning.

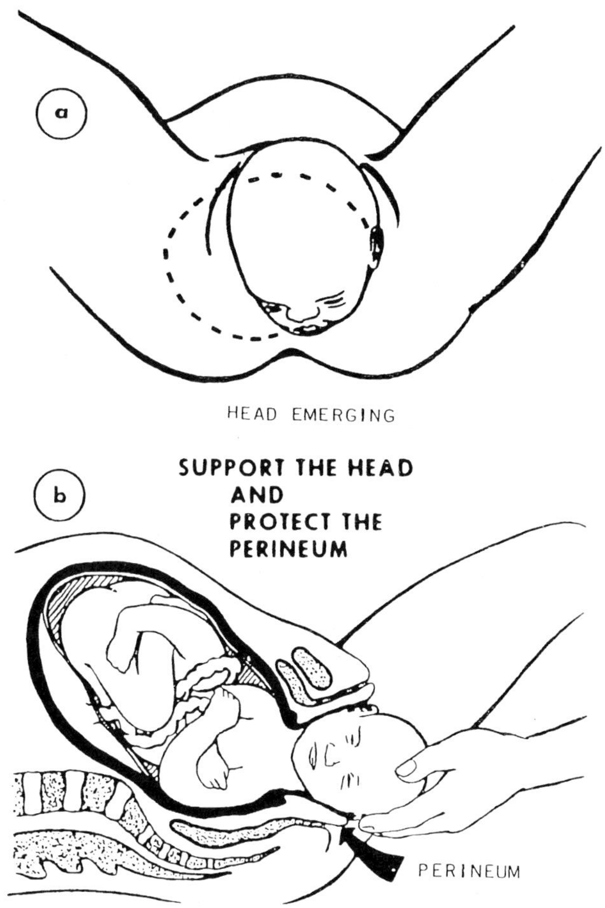

Figure 7–6. Second stage: support for head.

(5) Do not touch the vaginal area at any time.

(6) Put on sterile gloves, if available.

(7) Watch for emergence of the top of baby's head at the vagina. This is called crowning (fig. 7-5 (b)). Be prepared to support the baby's head as it emerges.

(8) As delivery is imminent (head crowning), get mother to pant with contractions. Permit the head to deliver between contractions, if at all possible. This will avoid perineal tears and trauma to infant's head by sudden release of pressure.

d. *Delivery of the Baby.*

(1) As the baby's head is born, it usually is face down; it then turns so that its nose is toward the mother's right or left thigh (fig. 7-6 (a)).

(2) Support the head by cradling it (fig. 7-6 (b) and fig. 7-7) between your hands. Do not pull or exert any pressure.

(3) To help the upper shoulder out, support the head in a downward position. To help the lower shoulder out, support the head in an upward position. As the shoulders emerge, be prepared for the rapid emergence of the rest of the baby's body—the head and shoulders are the widest parts and take longer to emerge.

(4) Use a sterile towel (or the cleanest article available) to receive the baby. Note the time, if possible, when the baby is born.

(5) As soon as it is completely delivered, pick the baby up to allow mucus and fluid to drain from its nose and mouth. Be sure you have a firm hold, as a newborn baby is very slippery. Grasp the baby at the ankles, slipping one of your fingers between them, and support shoulders with your other hand, with thumb and middle finger around neck and forefinger supporting the head (fig. 7-8).

(6) Do NOT pull on the cord when picking the baby up. Raise the baby's hips slightly higher than its head for drainage. It will probably breathe and cry almost immediately. Soon after this cry, the cord will become limp and will no longer pulsate. The blood flow ceases since the baby no longer needs it.

(7) If there seems to be excessive mucus, use your finger to clear the baby's mouth gently or use gentle suction with the rubber syringe. Support the baby by placing him on the mother's abdomen. The lowered head position can be maintained when clearing mucus by finger or syringe—do not attempt to support the baby in midair while holding it only by its feet.

(8) As soon as the baby is breathing and crying, wrap it in the blanket (if available). Do not pull on the cord. Do not tie the cord. The cord will usually be long enough for you to place the baby on the mother's abdomen. Help her to hold the baby there, in a side-lying position.

CONTROLLED DELIVERY OF THE HEAD

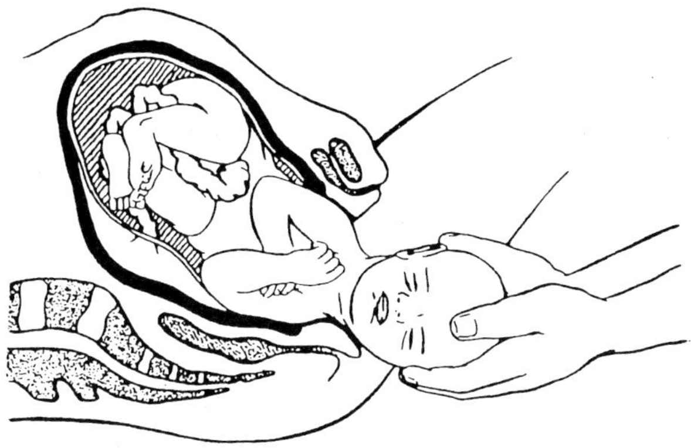

Figure 7-7. Second stage: cradling head between hands.

HOLDING THE BABY

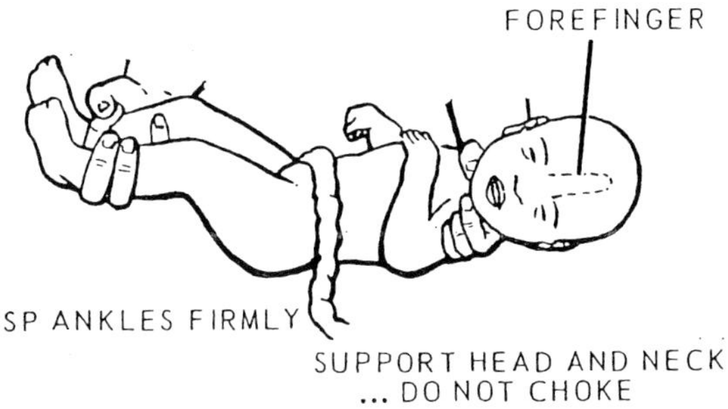

Figure 7-8. Holding the baby.

Delivery of the Placenta (Third Stage of Labor and Delivery)

a. Observe the appearance of the cord and its location at the vagina. As the placenta separates from the uterus, the cord will appear longer.

b. Place one hand on the mother's abdomen and feel for a definite contraction. The contracting uterus should feel like a hard, grapefruit-sized ball.

c. Wait for the delivery of the placenta. Ten minutes or longer will usually elapse before the placenta is delivered. Never pull on the cord to check for separation of the placenta. As the uterus contracts, encourage the mother to bear down to expel the placenta and membranes.

d. When the placenta appears at the vagina, grasp it gently and rotate it (fig. 7-9). Do not pull, but slowly and gently guide the placenta and attached membranes (fetal sac) from the mother's body.

e. Do not cut the cord. Wrap the placenta in a sterile towel. Place it next to the baby. Wrap the baby and placenta together in the third sterile sheet from the pack and place both in the mother's arms.

f. Check amount of vaginal bleeding. A small amount (one or two cups, or less than 500 ml) is expected.

g. Remove soiled sheet. Save all evidence of blood loss (stained sheet or towels) for doctor's examination.

h. Place two sanitary pads over vaginal and perineal area, touching only outer surface and placing from vaginal toward perineal area. Assist mother to place thighs together to hold pads in place.

i. Cover the mother and baby for warmth but do not overheat.

j. Check the baby's color and respirations. Encourage him to cry vigorously by gently flicking the soles of his feet with your finger.

k. Continue to check the feeling of hardness in the uterus. You should be able to cup your hands on either side of a firm hard ball about at the level of the mother's umbilicus (fig. 7-10). This is known as "guarding the fundus." If the fundus feels soft, use gentle massage to stimulate a firm hard contraction—this prevents bleeding.

l. Stay with the mother for at least one hour after delivery, unless relieved by competent personnel. The immediate postpartum period when hemorrhage may occur is dangerous for the mother. Check the fundus, her pulse and skin temperature. Watch for any signs of shock. Check vaginal pads for amount of bleeding without touching surface in contact with vagina.

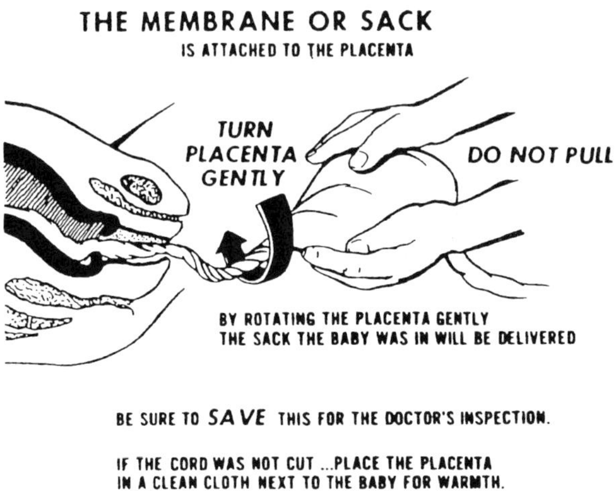

Figure 7–9. Delivery of placenta.

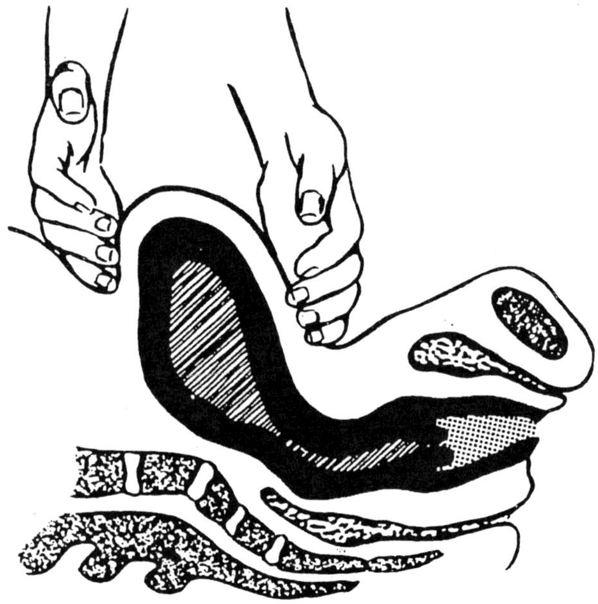

Figure 7–10. Third stage: checking fundus.

Special Points in Emergency Delivery

a. Avoid touching the vagina at any time, as there is great danger of infection.

b. Do not worry about tying the cord or cutting the cord. When the baby first cries, the circulation from baby to cord normally ceases, and clots form to seal off the umbilical blood vessels. The cord must only be cut under strict aseptic conditions because of possible infection. Leaving cord and placenta attached to the baby may be a bit messy, but it is safe.

c. Note time of birth and approximate location for legal registration.

d. If baby does not breathe spontaneously, clear mouth of mucus (fig. 7-11 (a)). Stimulate crying by gently rubbing back. If this fails, give extremely gentle mouth-to-mouth resuscitation. Hold head back, jaw up, and breathe gently into nose and mouth with small puffs—20 per minute (fig. 7-11 (b)).

e. If baby seems to have excessive amount of mucus after clearing its mouth, keep baby on side, in slight head-down position for gravity drainage. Turn baby from side to side to assist in aeration of lungs. Be extremely gentle when introducing your finger or the tip of the syringe into the baby's mouth.

f. If an unusual situation seems to be present—that is, the progress of labor and delivery seems other than described—

When in doubt, do nothing.
Get the mother to a hospital—fast.
Get medical advice by radio or telephone.

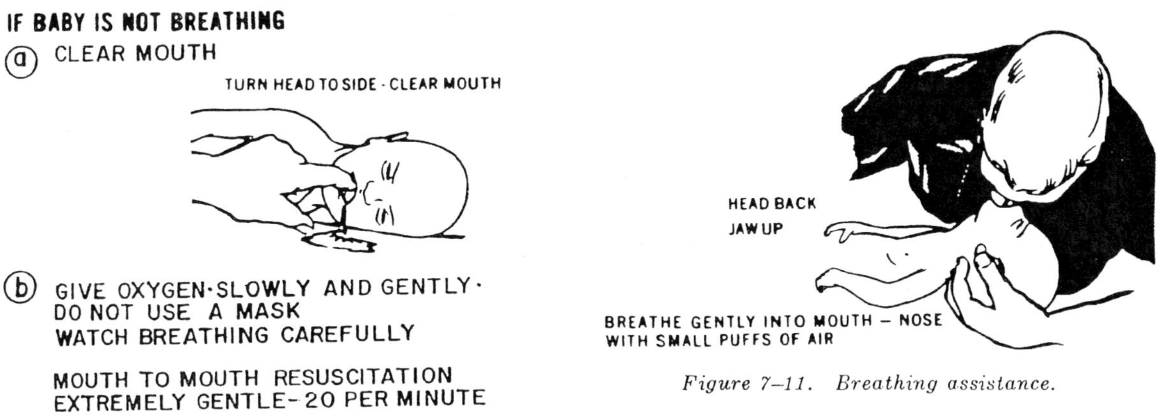

Figure 7–11. Breathing assistance.

Hospital Admission of Patient in Labor

NOTE:
The specialist in obstetrics will usually be female (WAC); the use of the term "he" is only for the purpose of continuity with the rest of the manual.

a. When a patient presents herself to the labor room, greet her cordially. If her husband is with her, instruct him where he can wait until the doctor evaluates the patient to see if she should be admitted. First impressions will frequently influence the patient's attitude and feelings throughout the labor and delivery process. As you prepare the patient for the doctor, obtain the following information:

- Contractions—onset, frequency, duration, length of time between.
- Bleeding, if any.

- Membranes ruptured or leakage of water from vagina.
- EDC.
- Number of pregnancies, number of live children.
- Time of last meal and whether she had anything to drink.

When a patient is ordered to be admitted to the ward, her prenatal record should be obtained. At this time also, the patient's temperature, pulse, respiration and blood pressure are taken and the fetal heart tones are checked. The operative permit for anesthetic and delivery should be signed.

b. After the patient is checked by the physician or the nurse and the status of labor established, a prep is done. Depending upon local policy, the pubic and perineal area or just the perineal area is prepped. If no contraindication, such as bleeding, rupture of membranes or advanced stage of labor is present, an enema is usually ordered. This will stimulate labor, evacuate the rectum and lessen the chance of contamination of the sterile field as the baby is delivered. A urine specimen is also obtained.

c. The specialist may be required to assist with the monitoring of the patient's progress as well as giving emotional support. The specialist will help time contractions, check the blood pressure and listen to the fetal heart tones. Any of the following must be reported to the nurse or physician immediately:

- Sudden increase or decrease in blood pressure
- Fetal heart tones below 120 or above 160 beats per minute
- Vaginal bleeding
- Rupture of membranes
- Impulse on part of mother to "push"

Emotional support includes staying with the patient as much as possible and making her as comfortable as possible. The specialist can sponge the patient's face and hands from time to time; give her ice chips (or a drink of water or tea with sugar, if not contraindicated); rub the lower part of her back; see that some fresh air is present; change her gown and/or bed linens if they get damp or soiled; and position patient on her side, if permitted.

Labor or Birth Complications

a. *Uterine Inertia:* Contractions so weak that they may cease entirely or be unable to force the baby out of the uterus.

b. *Precipitate Labor:* One that is very short with severe contractions. This may involve delivering the baby without a doctor and under unsterile conditions. Trauma can affect both mother and baby due to the severity of the labor.

c. *Abnormal Presentation:* Face, hand, foot or buttocks presented first, rather than the head.

d. *Cephalopelvic Disproportion:* Birth canal too small to permit the baby's head to pass through the pelvis.

e. *Cesarean Section:* A surgical procedure that involves removing the infant by making an incision in the abdomen and uterus. Repeat Cesarean sections are usually required in future births.

f. *Ruptured Uterus:* A rare condition in which the uterus splits from strain on the muscular wall due to severe labor contractions or to obstructed labor.

g. *Prolapsed Cord:* A serious complication in which circulation to the fetus is cut off and asphyxiation results. The umbilical cord may drop through the cervix after the membranes have ruptured. The cord may become compressed between the presenting part and the pelvic wall, thus cutting off fetal circulation.

h. *Toxemia:* A common condition in pregnancies (about one out of every 20). It occurs most frequently in the last months of pregnancy and is most likely to strike young women who are pregnant for the first time (primigravida) or women with a multiple pregnancy. Its symptoms can develop in a day or ever less, so the specialist must be ever vigilant and report immediately to the nurse or doctor any patient who shows any of the following symptoms:

- Sudden weight gain
- Blurred vision or spots before the eyes
- Edema of the face, fingers, legs or feet
- Decrease in urinary output
- Severe persistent headache
- Persistent vomiting
- Elevated blood pressure such as 140/90 or above
- Albumin in urine
- Mental confusion or disorientation

There are two stages of toxemia—

(1) *Preeclampsia:* A previously normal pregnant patient develops one or more of the symptoms.

(2) *Eclampsia:* In addition to any or all of the other symptoms, the patient has convulsions. Eclampsia can usually be prevented if the patient is carefully watched. Accurate observation and reporting are required because eclampsia is one of the most severe complications of pregnancy. Patients with eclampsia should be kept in a quiet room. Maternal mortality is from 5% to 15%; fetal mortality is about 25%.

i. *Fetal Distress:* This is indicated by a change in fetal heart tones (either an increase to above 160 beats/minute or a decrease below 100 beats/minute), rapid excessive movements of the fetus, and/or the presence of meconium in the vaginal discharge when the presenting part is the head. Fetal distress may result from premature labor, prolapsed umbilical cord, toxemia or hemorrhage due to placenta previa (note 1) or to placenta abruptio (note 2). When this condition occurs, labor may be started early, or an unexpected Cesarean section may have to be done. In the latter instance, the specialist must move rapidly to get the needed equipment ready.

NOTE 1

There are three types of placenta previa (painless bleeding)—

(1) Centralis—placenta has been implanted in the lower uterine segment and completely covers the cervix.

(2) Lateral—placenta lies in the lower uterine segment but does not cover any part of the cervix.

(3) Marginal—placenta partially covers the cervix.

NOTE 2

Placenta abruptio is a condition in which the placenta prematurely separates from the uterine wall. Patients with this condition have a painful, rigid abdomen with no visible bleeding.

j. *Other Complications.* These include hemorrhage and severe chronic disease in the patient.

Post Partum Care of Mother

The mother is observed closely for several hours after delivery. Since she is often chilled, a blanket should be readily available. The first hour of post partum is the most critical one for the mother. It is during this time that post partum hemorrhage is most likely to occur as a result of uterine relaxation. The fundus should be checked at least every 15 minutes. In those patients whose uterus tends to relax, the fundus should be watched almost constantly. Firm massage over the fundus helps the uterus contract to a firm mass about the size of a grapefruit. The fundus is usually slightly below the umbilicus unless the bladder is full. Check pads for amount of bleeding. Pulse, blood pressure and distention of bladder must be checked frequently during this period. The following should be observed during the post partum period:

a. *Lochia.* This is a normal vaginal discharge consisting of blood and lining from the uterus which occurs in diminishing amounts in the early post partum period. The first 3 to 4 days, the lochia is bloodstained. Gradually, the color becomes brownish, and by the tenth day, the discharge is usually a yellowish-white. A foul odor to the lochia may be an indication of interuterine infection. The presence of blood in the lochia after the tenth day is abnormal. In both of these instances, the doctor should be immediately notified.

b. *After Pains.* Painful cramps may occur as the uterine muscles contract. This is especially noticeable when patient is nursing the infant. This usually occurs in multipara patients and lasts 3 to 4 days.

c. *Bladder.* This should be observed for distention as it may become distended without any awareness by the patient. Patient must void or be catheterized q. 6-8 hours. If the fundus remains above the umbilicus and cannot be massaged down, it is a good indication that the bladder is full. To check the amount of urine in the bladder, measure area between bottom of fundus and pubic arch. The bladder should be checked by palpation after voiding to be sure it is empty. Frequently, muscle tone of the bladder is lost for varying periods after delivery and there is retention of urine.

d. Breasts. A good supportive brassiere should be worn day and night from the first day after delivery whether the mother plans to breast feed or not. If not breast feeding, and depending upon local policy, a lactation prevention medication may be given at time of delivery. Support and normal hygiene is usually all that is necessary. When the milk starts coming in (2-3 days after delivery), engorgement (hardness of breasts) may occur in some women. This usually disappears in about 24 hours. DO NOT stimulate the breasts by expressing the milk; leave alone. If the mother is breast feeding, a good nursing brassiere should be worn day and night. Since the procedures for cleaning the nipples and teaching mother and baby how to breast feed vary widely, check with the nurse or the physician in each instance.

e. Perineal Area. All patients receive perineal care; however, if the patient has had an episiotomy (incision in the perineum during delivery), she must be exposed to thermolite treatments (gooseneck lamp or patient's bed lamp with a no stronger than 40-watt bulb which is placed 10-12 inches from the perineum) several times daily to insure that the area is kept clean and dry. In any perineal care, cleansing is accomplished from the pubic area toward the rectum to avoid contamination with feces. Fresh tissues are used for each stroke.

f. Early Ambulation. In most hospitals the doctor will want the mother up 4 to 6 hours after delivery, depending on the anesthesia given during delivery. The specialist should get the patient up slowly to prevent dizziness and assist on the first trip to the bathroom (remaining with the patient) and as often afterwards as necessary.

g. Bathing. The patient has a daily bath or shower, as the doctor orders.

h. Exercises. A routine system of simple exercises designed to tighten muscles overstretched during pregnancy and to correct basic posture can be started 24 hours after delivery. These exercises are frequently taught by the physical therapy section.

Immediate Care of Baby

a. After the physician has finished working with the baby (this usually includes suctioning the respiratory tract, clamping and cutting the umbilical cord and instilling medication in the eyes to prevent possible gonorrheal infection, although the nurse may do the latter), he hands the baby to the nurse who has a warm blanket and bassinet ready. During this time and afterward, there must be a *constant observation* of the baby for any respiratory distress and excessive mucus, which would necessitate immediate suctioning. Resuscitation tray with endotracheal tube and laryngoscope must always be available if needed by doctor. An APGAR score is noted by the nurse or physician at one minute after birth. The APGAR "score" or scale is an aid in making an evaluation of the success and the speed of the newborn's initial adjustment to extra-uterine living. Five signs are evaluated and scored as indicated in table 7-1. The total score of the five signs is 8 to 10 when initial adjustment is good. Lower scores require special attention.

b. Before the newborn is taken from the delivery room, the nurse or specialist must apply identification bands to both wrists or ankles. These bands show mother's name, infant's sex, date, time of birth, doctor's name and mother's register number.

c. If the baby is in poor condition and the parent's religion requires baptism, immediate arrangements should be made. Anyone can baptize, but the form is important and a record should be made on the mother's chart, along with the name of two witnesses, whenever possible. If a nurse or a specialist must baptize a baby, this procedure should be followed:

(1) Pour a small amount of water on the baby's face or forehead.

(2) While pouring, say "I baptize you in the name of the Father and of the Son and of the Holy Ghost (Spirit)," or if the baby may be dead, "If you are alive, I baptize you in the name of the Father and of the Son and of the Holy Ghost (Spirit)."

Table 7-1. APGAR Scale for Evaluating Condition of the Newborn

Sign	Score		
	0	1	2
Heart rate	Absent	Slow, below 100	Over 100
Respiratory rate	Absent	Slow, irregular	Good cry
Muscle tone	Limp	Flexion of arms or legs	Active motion
Reflex instability*	No response	Grimace	Cough or sneeze
Color	All blue or all pale	Body pink, extremities blue	Completely pink

*Tested by insertion of catheter tip into nostril.

Table 7-2. Policies for Newborn Nursery

DO—	DO NOT—
Clean nursery by wet mopping several times a day	Do NOT use curtains or any other type of dust-catcher in the nursery.
Wipe *all* equipment with disinfectant *every* day.	
If authorized to enter the nursery, report to the nurse in charge if you have any sore throat, skin infection, or any other infectious condition.	•Do NOT permit unauthorized personnel to enter the nursery.
Scrub hands for 5 minutes when reporting on duty or after using latrine.	
Move around the nursery and check each unit, as constant vigilance is required. Prematures need closer observations than normal infants.	•Do NOT give information about infants to anyone except the parents or as directed by the nurse.
Wash hands thoroughly before touching an infant	•Do NOT go from one infant to another without washing your hands.
Provide each infant with his own crib and stock of supplies	•Do NOT use the same equipment for two infants.
Place soiled diapers in step-on cans with lids and remove from the nursery periodically.	•Do NOT put soiled diapers on the infant's crib or on the floor.
Autoclave any linen coming into the nursery.	
Change from uniform to scrub suit in the nursery dressing room. Caps and masks may be required.	

Newborn Nursery

Infants born in the hospital are normally admitted to the nursery. The important policies in table 7-2 that maintain cleanliness and reduce contamination for protection of the babies are a "must" in this area.

General Care for Newborns

a. Observation. The infant is observed for—

(1) Cyanosis
(2) Hemorrhage
(3) Rapid, labored, grunting respirations
(4) Vomiting or choking
(5) Redness or discharge from eyes
(6) Redness around the cord
(7) Thrush (redness of tongue and mucous membranes of the mouth and closely adherent white patches)
(8) Diarrhea
(9) Jaundice
(10) Rash of any kind
(11) Temperature elevation
(12) Failure to pass meconium 12 hours after birth or failure to urinate

b. Identification Band. This band must be checked each time the baby is given to its mother or to the nurse. Bands for premature infants are usually taped to the isolette and placed on the baby when it has attained added weight.

c. Other Identification. Palm or footprints of the baby and the mother's fingerprints may be taken as an added precaution.

d. Measurements. Infant is weighed, length is measured, and circumference of head and chest is measured. Infant must be protected from chilling during these procedures.

e. Skin Care. In most nurseries, babies are *lightly* washed with hexachlorophene and water and cotton sponges. Some of the vernix caseosa (a greasy white, cheesy-like substance covering the baby at birth) will remain, particularly on the head, but will gradually absorb and wear off. Any gross blood is removed the same way.

WARNING
Gauze or terry washcloths must *not* be used, as they will irritate the baby's skin.

The buttocks are cleaned the same way, rubbing as little as possible. The eyes are washed with sterile water.

f. Cord Care. The area around the cord must be kept clean. Dressings are *not* added unless the doctor orders. The cord is usually swabbed with a solution of 70% alcohol or hexachlorophene.

g. Temperature. A separate thermometer is used for each infant. Rectal temperature is taken on admission to the nursery and every 4 hours until stabilized; thereafter, it is taken only once a day. The temperature usually drops to 96°F after birth, then gradually climbs to 98°F or 99°F. Any deviation should be reported. Depending upon your local policy, the infant is placed in an incubator if the temperature is below 97.6°F until temperature rises.

h. Elimination. The time the baby first voids should be recorded, as well as the character (usually clear), and the time of the first stool, which will be composed of *meconium* (tarry green substance). The number and type of bowel movements thereafter should also be recorded. Mucus, blood or curds in the stool should be recorded at once.

i. Feedings—Newborn Infant

(1) The normal newborn is kept NPO the first 12 hours or as ordered, then given a preparation of glucose water for the first two feedings. After the glucose water, the infant is fed by breast, or a prescribed formula is given every 4 hours.

(2) The premature infant is kept NPO the first 24 hours or as ordered, and then given a preparation of glucose water or a formula feeding as prescribed by the pediatrician.

j. Weighing. In the newborn nursery, newborns are usually weighed daily, or as determined by local policy. The scale used should be properly balanced; the time of weighing approximately the same for each day; and allowances made for pads, diapers or clothing which are weighed with the infant.

OBSTETRIC AND GYNECOLOGIC EMERGENCIES

OBSTETRIC AND GYNECOLOGIC EMERGENCIES

Unit 1. Anatomy and Physiology of the Female Reproductive System

In this unit, the basic functions and anatomical structures of the female reproductive system will be summarized, as will the developmental stages of pregnancy and the progression of normal labor and delivery.

Anatomy

The female reproductive system includes the ovaries, fallopian tubes, uterus, and vagina. The female reproductive organs are located in the pelvic cavity. The uterus lies above and behind the bladder. The bladder orifice, the urethra, opens in front of the vaginal opening. The rectum and its opening, the anus, lie behind the vagina. The vaginal, urethral, and rectal orifices open into a region called the perineum. Because these pelvic organs lie so close to the uterus and vagina, trauma to the reproductive organs also can injure the bladder, urethra, rectum, or anus.

Ovaries. The ovaries are two walnut-shaped organs located in the right and left lower quadrants. These organs produce ova (eggs). Progesterone and estrogen, the female sex hormones, also are produced by the ovaries. In the nonpregnant woman, estrogen and progesterone secretion varies cyclically each month. In the pregnant woman, estrogen and progesterone secretion varies according to the stage of pregnancy. Two hormones secreted by the anterior pituitary gland, follicle-stimulating hormone and luteinizing hormone, regulate ovarian hormone secretion.

Estrogen thickens the linings of the uterus (endometrium), fallopian tubes, and vagina. In addition, estrogen produces female secondary sexual characteristics. Estrogen also affects kidney function. It decreases sodium, chloride, and water excretion, thereby decreasing urine output and increasing extracellular fluid volume.

Progesterone can act only on tissues that have been primed by estrogen. Progesterone prepares the reproductive tract for implantation of a fertilized egg. It also prepares the breast for lactation (milk production). Body temperature is slightly increased (0.5° to 1.0° F) by progesterone secretion.

The ovaries release one mature ovum about once a month during the reproductive years. Since the ovaries are not directly connected to the fallopian tubes, the ova enter the peritoneal cavity before being drawn into the fallopian tubes.

Fallopian tubes. The fallopian tubes allow the passage of the ova from the ovaries to the uterus. At their ovarian ends, the fallopian tubes are funnel shaped and fringed with small fingerlike structures called fimbria that insure that ova reach the fallopian tubes from the ovaries. At their uterine ends, the fallopian tubes are narrower.

Uterus cervix and vagina The ovum travels through the fallopian tube into a pear-shaped, muscular organ called the uterus (womb). In the nonpregnant woman, the uterus is about 3 inches high, 2 inches wide, and 1 inch thick. It is located above and behind the bladder. In the pregnant woman, the uterus enlarges and rises upward. By the end of pregnancy, the uterus is 12 inches high, 9 inches wide, and 8 inches thick.

The uterus has three layers: the perimetrium, the myometrium, and the endometrium. The perimetrium is the peritoneal covering of the uterus that separates it from the abdominal cavity. The myometrium is a thick, muscular layer that forms most of the uterine wall. The endometrium is the inner lining of the uterus. Its thickness varies cyclically each month in nonpregnant women.

During the early part of the menstrual cycle, the endometrium thickens to prepare for ovulation (release of a mature ovum). If the ovum is fertilized by uniting with a sperm cell, it will implant in the endometrium and develop into a fetus. If the ovum is not fertilized, however, the uterus sheds its endometrial lining 14 days after ovulation. Shedding of the endometrial lining produces a menstrual period, during which there is a discharge of a bloody fluid from the uterus. Menstrual periods occur about every 28 days and last 3 to 7 days during the reproductive years. Menstrual periods are absent, of course, during pregnancy.

At the distal end of the uterus is a narrow opening called the cervix, through which the menstrual flow passes and through which the fetus passes during labor and delivery. The cervix connects the uterus to the vagina. The vagina is a muscular tube leading to the external genitalia. The vagina serves as the birth canal during labor and delivery.

The ovaries, fallopian tubes, uterus, and vagina receive blood from the ovarian, uterine, and vaginal arteries. The ovarian arteries arise from the aorta, just below the origins of the renal arteries. These arteries supply the ovaries, fallopian tubes, and part of the uterus. The uterine arteries mainly supply the uterus. The vaginal arteries mainly supply the vagina. Because the blood supply to the internal reproductive organs is complex bleeding from these organs may be extensive and fatal if untreated.

The external female genitalia include the vulval structures external to the reproductive organs. The vulval structures include the labia majora and the labia minora. The labia majors are large, rounded, lateral skin folds. These enlarge as they pass forward from the anus and meet at the symphysis pubis. (The symphysis pubis is the anterior joint between the two pubic bones that form part of the pelvic girdle.) The labia minora are smaller skin folds that are medial to the labia majora and usually are hidden by them.

The breasts are secretory glands located on the anterior chest wall. During pregnancy, estrogen and progesterone act on the breasts to prepare them for lactation following delivery. After delivery, prolactin and oxytocin, hormones secreted by the pituitary gland, stimulate the breasts to produce milk.

Pregnancy

Pregnancy begins when an ovum unites with a sperm cell that has been introduced into the female reproductive tract. Union of the ovum and sperm cell is called fertilization and occurs in the fallopian tube. The fertilized ovum then passes into the uterus and implants in the endometrium. Implantation usually occurs in the upper part of the uterus.

The fertilized ovum develops into a fetus. The fetus is nourished by the placenta. The placenta, a special disk-shaped organ, develops during pregnancy and attaches to the inner wall of the uterus. The placenta contains both fetal and maternal tissues. Oxygen and nutrients diffuse from the maternal bloodstream into the fetal bloodstream through the placenta. Carbon dioxide and waste products also diffuse from the fetal blood vessels into the maternal blood vessels through the placenta. Maternal and fetal blood vessels are in close contact with the placenta, but the two bloodstreams do not mix.

Fetal blood enters and leaves the placenta through blood vessels contained in the umbilical cord. These umbilical vessels enter the fetus through the umbilicus, or navel. Two umbilical arteries carry unoxygenated blood from the fetus to the placenta. A single umbilical vein returns oxygenated blood to the fetus.

The combined blood flow into the placenta from the fetal and maternal circulation is large in volume. Therefore, any disturbance to the placenta (e.g., separation from the uterine wall or change in position) will cause extensive bleeding and endanger both the fetus and the mother. In addition, blood supply to the entire uterus increases during pregnancy. Therefore uterine injuries also can produce extensive bleeding

During development in the uterus, the fetus is enclosed in the amniotic sac (bag of waters). This sac contains amniotic fluid in which the fetus floats freely. The amniotic fluid helps protect the fetus from mechanical injury. Amniotic fluid is formed from maternal serum and fetal urine; it is reabsorbed into the maternal circulation and also swallowed by the fetus. At the end of pregnancy, the amniotic sac contains about 1 liter (1) of amniotic fluid. During or before labor, this sac ruptures, and amniotic fluid flows out through the cervix and the vagina.

Physiologic changes characteristic of pregnancy are used to determine whether a woman is pregnant and when she will give birth. Pregnancy begins when the ovum is fertilized by a sperm cell, usually about 14 days after the beginning of the last menstrual period. Although it is impossible to determine exactly when fertilization actually occurs, it is easy to determine when the last menstrual period began. For this reason, duration of pregnancy is usually determined by assuming that pregnancy began on the first day of the last menstrual period. Each 4-week period of pregnancy is called a lunar month. There are 10 lunar months in a normal pregnancy. Each 3-month period is called a trimester.

During the first 4 weeks of pregnancy (1st lunar month), the pregnant woman stops menstruating, her breasts enlarge, and she sleeps more than usual. In addition, she urinates more frequently because the pregnant uterus presses on the bladder.

From the 5th through the 8th week (2d lunar month), she may experience nausea and vomiting in addition to the above symptoms. In the 9th through 12th weeks of pregnancy (3d lunar month), the uterus can be felt above the symphysis pubis, and urinary frequency returns to normal. Between the 13th and 16th weeks (4th lunar month), the pregnant woman begins to feel fetal movement.

Between the 17th and 20th weeks (5th lunar month), fetal heart sounds can be heard with a stethoscope. By the end of the 24th week (6th lunar month), the examiner can feel fetal movement.

During the 37th through the 40th week (10th lunar month), the uterus drops back down as the presenting part descends into the pelvis. The uterus presses on the bladder, and urinary frequency again increases.

Labor is the process during which the uterus repeatedly contracts to push the fetus and placenta out of the mother's body. Delivery is the actual birth of the baby at the end of the second stage of labor.

Before labor begins, the head of the fetus settles in the pelvis. The cervix then begins to efface, or thin. Effacement may be completed before labor begins or may continue during the first stage of labor.

At the beginning of labor, contractions are far apart. As labor progresses, contractions occur closer together. During the most active stage of labor, contractions occur every 2 to 3 minutes and last 30 to 45 seconds.

There are three stages of labor. The first stage begins with the first uterine contraction and lasts until the cervix is completely effaced and dilated (open). A completely dilated cervix is about 10 centimeters wide. The first stage usually lasts about 12 hours in a woman who has previously borne a child. The amniotic sac frequently ruptures when the cervix is completely dilated.

The second stage of labor begins when the fetus starts descending into the vagina. Normally, the head descends first; this type of delivery is called cephalic (head). If the buttocks descend first, it is called a breech delivery. During the second stage of labor, the woman will bear down with each contraction. As the presenting part of the fetus presses on the rectum, the woman will feel an urge to defecate. The presenting part will appear at the vaginal opening during each contraction and disappear again between contractions. Eventually, the presenting part will remain visible between contractions. This is called crowning. In a normal delivery, the head will then be born and the shoulders and trunk will be born soon after the head. The second stage of labor usually lasts about an hour in a woman having a first baby and from 15 to 20 minutes in a woman who has previously borne a child.

In the third stage of labor, uterine contractions expel the placenta. When the placenta separates from the uterine wall, a small amount of blood gushes out through the vagina. Then, the placenta is pushed out of the uterus and through the vagina. The third stage of labor usually lasts about 15 minutes.

Unit 2. Pathophysiology and Management of Gynecologic Emergencies

In general, there is little that paramedics can do to treat gynecologic emergencies in the field. Most common gynecologic emergencies require the attention of a physician or the use of specialized treatment resources not found in the emergency vehicle. However, the paramedic can greatly aid the physician and the hospital staff by obtaining an adequate history from the patient.

Abdominal Pain

A gynecologic problem, that is, a problem related to the female reproductive organs, should be suspected in any woman who presents with abdominal pain. The following questions should be asked to obtain information necessary for possible future treatment:

- When was the patient's last menstrual period? Was it unusual in any way? Has she had any bleeding between menstrual periods or bleeding following menopause?
- Has she missed a menstrual period? Does she use any form of contraception? Could she be pregnant?
- Has she had any vaginal discharge? What color was it? Was it foul smelling?
- Where is the pain exactly? What is it like (sharp, dull, constant, intermittent)? What makes it better? What makes it worse? Is it made worse by sexual intercourse? Row long has it been between the onset of the pain and the last menstrual period?

Pelvic inflammatory disease (PID). Often resulting from gonorrhea, PID is one of the most common sources of abdominal pain in women. The pain is sometimes diffuse but sometimes is localized to one of the lower quadrants. It may radiate to the right shoulder and is often quite severe. In many cases, the pain begins at about the time of the menstrual period. It may be accompanied by fever, nausea, and vomiting. The pain frequently is made worse by sexual intercourse. The patient usually complains of moderate to heavy vaginal discharge. The patient's recent menstrual history often is characterized by missed periods and by bleeding between periods.

Physical examination often reveals a very ill-appearing patient. In general, blood pressure is normal, and pulse is elevated. Fever may be present. Palpation of the abdomen causes moderate to extreme pain and should be done very gently. No treatment in the field is necessary for patients with PID. Such patients should be made comfortable in whatever position they prefer and transported gently to the hospital.

Other sources of abdominal pain. Other possible sources of abdominal pain in women include ectopic pregnancy (i.e., the fetus growing in a location outside of the uterus, e.g., in the fallopian tube), ruptured ovarian cyst, and nongynecologic causes such as appendicitis and cystitis (bladder inflammation). Differentiating these conditions in the field is not vitally important, as management for most consists of support and transport of the patient. Ectopic pregnancies, however, must be distinguished from other causes of abdominal pain as they can lead to hypovolemic shock. Recognition and treatment of ruptured ectopic pregnancies will be discussed in Unit 3 of this chapter.

Vaginal Bleeding

Vaginal bleeding may follow trauma or may occur in the absence of trauma. General management of abnormal vaginal bleeding will be discussed in the following section.

Vaginal bleeding with no history of trauma. In questioning the patient who complains of vaginal bleeding, it is important for the paramedic to try to estimate the amount of blood lost. What may seem like an alarming amount to the patient may be clinically insignificant. The patient should be asked how long she has been bleeding and how many sanitary napkins she has used. The paramedic should determine whether the bleeding has been heavier or lighter than that during a normal menstrual period, as well as what the patient has used to absorb the blood (towels generally soak up less blood than a sanitary napkin). Blood loss can be assessed further in the physical exam by checking for variations in pulse rate due to a change in posture. An increase in pulse rate of more than 20 per minute when the patient goes from a supine to a sitting position is highly suggestive of blood loss greater than one unit. If this finding is positive, the paramedic should treat the patient like any other patient in impending shock by:

- Administering oxygen
- Placing the patient supine with the legs slightly elevated
- Starting an intravenous (Iv) line with normal saline or Ringer's solution and infusing it rapidly
- Following vital signs closely en route to the hospital

Vaginal bleeding accompanied by genital trauma. Rape or other trauma may result in lacerations of the external female genitalia. Lacerations may be accompanied by heavy bleeding. Usually this bleeding can be controlled simply by applying external pressure over the laceration. Bleeding from the internal genitalia can be massive. It is both useless and dangerous to introduce packs blindly into the vagina in an attempt to control bleeding. A pack should be used only if bleeding is life threatening, in which case a sterile towel or sterile 2-inch gauze tape should be tightly packed into the vagina. The Military Anti-Shock Trousers (MAST) apparatus will probably not help control bleeding from the internal genitalia but will provide an autotransfusion effect of approximately two units and, therefore, should be applied. As in any case of massive hemorrhage, the patient with severe vaginal bleeding needs at least one and preferably two or three IV lines for rapid infusion of normal saline, Ringer's solution, or a plasma derivative. Other standard measures for shock apply here as well. Vital signs must be monitored minute by minute and transport to the hospital should be rapid.

Caring for the Rape Victim

Rape presents a difficult and complex problem, involving physical and emotional trauma as well as potential legal ramifications. It is essential that a good history be obtained from the rape victim. In questioning the patient, the paramedic must use tact and sensitivity. The patient may find it extremely difficult to discuss what has happened and may fear, or feel hostile toward, a male paramedic. Every effort should be made to understand the patient's feelings and to respond with kindness and reassurance. The emotional trauma of rape is usually more prolonged and severe than the physical trauma. The attitude shown toward the patient during her care can have a serious influence, for good or ill, on her future psychological and physical recovery.

A primary assessment should be conducted for the rape victim, as for any other patient. The paramedic should observe whether the patient's clothes are torn or in disarray. The paramedic also should check for trauma elsewhere on the patient's body, especially around the thighs, lower abdomen, and buttocks. If vaginal bleeding is significant, it should be treated as outlined earlier.

The report submitted by the paramedic to the emergency department should state only what the patient said, in her own words, and what the paramedic observed. The paramedic's opinion as to whether the patient was raped should not be included in the report. Every rape is a potential court case, and the report is a legal document. Therefore, the paramedic should be thorough and accurate.

Unit 3. Pathophysiology and Management of Obstetric Emergencies

Emergency obstetrics situations in which the paramedic will be likely to become involved include normal labor and delivery, complications of labor and delivery, and conditions that can be life threatening to the pregnant woman or to the fetus before labor.

Serious medical problems that the pregnant woman may encounter before labor are termed antepartum complications. In this unit, several types of antepartum complications will be discussed: five conditions involving hemorrhage and several other conditions involving supine hypotensive syndrome and toxemia.

Antepartum Hemorrhage Complications

Hemorrhage complications occurring before delivery are classified as antepartum complications. Five antepartum hemorrhage conditions will be discussed in this section: abortion, ectopic pregnancy, abruptio placentae, placenta previa, and uterine rupture.

Abortion. Abortion is defined as loss of pregnancy before the 20th week of gestation (the 20th week of fetal growth). It often is referred to by laypeople as a "miscarriage." Abortions can occur spontaneously or can be induced. Induced abortions that are performed under sterile conditions in authorized medical settings are termed therapeutic abortions. Abortions that occur naturally fall into one of the four categories discussed below.

Threatened abortion.--Signs and symptoms of threatened abortion include vaginal bleeding, pain resembling menstrual cramps, and, occasionally, dilation of the cervix. This condition can progress to complete abortion or may subside, and the pregnancy may go to term. A woman with a threatened abortion should be evaluated at the hospital. Treatment is bed rest.

Inevitable abortion.--An abortion that cannot be prevented is termed an inevitable abortion. Signs of an impending abortion include vaginal bleeding, which can be very heavy, uterine contractions, and cervical dilation. For a patient with such symptoms, the paramedic should start an IV with normal saline or Ringer's solution. She should be transported to the hospital as quickly as possible. Fluids should be given as rapidly as possible to maintain blood pressure during transport.

Incomplete abortion.--An incomplete abortion occurs when part of the fetus is expelled and part of the products of conception remain within the uterus. This situation causes hemorrhage and continued cervical dilation. The patient should be treated for shock if it is present. Products of conception protruding from the cervix should be gently removed to prevent sepsis. Paramedics should consult the physician for instructions in treating a patient with an incomplete abortion.

Missed abortion.--In a missed abortion, the fetus dies before 20-weeks gestation but is retained in the uterus for at least 2 months following death. The uterus hardens, and fetal heart sounds are no longer present. The patient with a missed abortion should be taken to the hospital for further treatment.

Ectopic pregnancy. The fertilized ovum may implant abnormally in the fallopian tube, ovary, or abdomen, rather than in the uterus. Implantation in the fallopian tube (tubal pregnancy) is far more coon than implantation in either the ovary or the abdomen; such a condition is very rare. Ectopic pregnancy is also 10 times more frequent in women who become pregnant with an IUD in place.

Fertilization normally occurs in the fallopian tubes. In a tubal pregnancy, the fertilized ovum fails to travel into the uterus and is implanted in the fallopian tube. Abnormalities of either the ovum or the fallopian tubes can prevent the ovum from reaching the uterus. Tubal abnormalities can result from developmental defects, previous infection and scarring, as in pelvic inflammatory disease, or cancer involving the tube.

When the fertilized ovum implants in the muscular layer of the fallopian tube, it invades maternal blood vessels. The fallopian tube does not enlarge as the fetus grows, and the tube eventually ruptures. This rupture may be either internal into the tube lumen or external into the abdominal cavity, and the resulting blood loss may be entirely hidden.

The patient with a ruptured tubal pregnancy complains of severe pain localized to one lower quadrant. She may have vaginal bleeding. If blood enters the abdominal cavity, it will irritate the peritoneum and cause fever. The accumulated blood produces a mass that is tender to palpation.

As blood loss continues, hypovolemic shock develops. The pulse becomes rapid; and the skin becomes pale, cold, and moist. When the body can no longer compensate for the decreased blood volume, the blood pressure falls.

Hypovolemic shock due to ruptured ectopic pregnancy should be treated in the same way as hypovolemic shock due to other causes. To treat hypovolemic shock, the paramedic should:

- Administer oxygen
- Support ventilation, if necessary
- Take vital signs
- Apply and inflate the MAST
- Start two or more large-bore (14- to 16-gauge) IV lines, and then rapidly infuse normal saline, Ringer's solution, or a plasma derivative
- Place the patient in supine position with feet elevated 300
- Keep patient warm
- Monitor state of consciousness, pulse, and blood pressure during transport

Abruptio placentae. Abruptio placentae occurs when a normally implanted placenta separates prematurely from the uterine wall during the last trimester of pregnancy. The patient experiences severe lower abdominal pain, and the uterus becomes rigid. Shock may be more severe than the apparent blood loss would seem to indicate.

Placenta previa. Placenta previa is a condition in which the placenta, rather than the baby, is the presenting part. This condition also occurs in the third trimester. Again, hemorrhage may be severe from the highly vascular placental tissue. Pain is frequently absent in this disorder.

Uterine rupture. Uterine rupture is manifested by sudden, severe abdominal pain. Bleeding may not be apparent externally, but profound shock can occur from internal hemorrhage.

To treat the patient for shock, the paramedic should:

- Place the patient horizontally on a stretcher, preferably on her side
- Administer oxygen
- Apply the MAST to produce autotransfusion
- Start at least two large-bore IV lines, and administer 50-percent dextrose in normal saline (D5NS), D5W dextrose in Ringer's solution, or a plasma derivative as rapidly as needed to maintain blood pressure
- Transport the patient to the hospital

Other Antepartum Conditions

The paramedic may also encounter other serious antepartum conditions such as supine hypotensive syndrome and toxemia.

Supine hypotensive syndrome. The pregnant woman near term has a large, heavy mass in her abdomen. When she is supine, this mass, which includes the weight of the uterus, fetus, and placenta, tends to compress the inferior vena cava. Venous return to the heart is thereby reduced, and, as a result, cardiac output falls. These changes are especially pronounced when the mother's vascular volume is low to begin with, as, for example, in antepartum hemorrhage. When a pregnant patient near term who is hypotensive or complains of dizziness is encountered, she should be placed on her side. Severe hypotension indicates a possibility of significant internal hemorrhage. Severe hypotension should be treated like hypovolemic shock as discussed above.

Toxemia of pregnancy. Toxemia of pregnancy has two stages: preeclampsia and eclampsia. Preeclampsia is characterized by hypertension (blood pressure greater than 140/90), proteinuria (protein in the urine), and edema during the last 3 months of pregnancy. Eclampsia follows preeclampsia and includes convulsions and/or coma in addition to the signs of preeclampsia.

In preeclampsia, renal blood flow and glomerular filtration are below the normal level for pregnant women. Thus, urine output and sodium excretion decrease. This condition increases extracellular fluid volume and produces edema in the ankles, fingers, and face.

Other symptoms of preeclampsia are headache, mid-upper abdominal pain, and blurred vision. Elevated blood pressure and edema, however, are necessary for a diagnosis of preeclampsia. Therefore, the paramedic should report the blood pressure and the presence or absence of edema in every pregnant woman examined for any complaint.

The patient with preeclampsia should be evaluated by a physician in the emergency department and will probably require hospitalization. When transporting the patient, the paramedic should remember that preeclampsia can progress to eclampsia with convulsions and/or coma and should be prepared to treat these.

Eclampsia can occur before, during, or after labor. It begins with convulsions that are usually followed by coma. The eclamptic patient, like the preeclamptic patient, has pronounced hypertension and edema. Her urine will be scant and bloody. She also may show signs and symptoms of pulmonary edema.

Although the physician should be contacted for specific directions in treating eclampsia, the paramedic can do the following:

- Establish and maintain an airway; administer oxygen.
- Start an IV with D5W to keep open. Do not use normal saline or Ringer's solution as they will increase the fluid overload.
- If convulsions occur and the physician orders diazepam (Valium), administer 5-10 milligrams (mg) slowly IV; if 10-percent magnesium sulfate is ordered, administer 2-4 mg slowly IV.
- Administer furosemide (Lasix) to reduce extracellular fluid volume, if ordered by the physician.
- Transport the patient gently to the hospital without flashing red lights or sirens, as these can cause convulsions.

In antepartum hemorrhage of any kind, the paramedic should <u>not attempt to examine the patient internally.</u>

<u>Normal Delivery</u>

Assisting in the birth of a baby, bringing life into the world, is one of the few situations in which the paramedic will have the opportunity to participate in a happy event, rather than an unpleasant one. The situation is also unique in that the paramedic is dealing with two patients, the mother and the baby, both of whom require skilled attention.

When paramedics arrive at the scene of a woman in labor, they first will need to determine whether there is time to transport the patient to the hospital. To make this decision, the paramedic should answer the following questions:

- Has the mother had a baby before? Labor during a first pregnancy is usually slower than in subsequent pregnancies; therefore, there may be more time for transport during a first labor.
- How frequent are the contractions? Contractions more than 5 minutes apart are a good indication that there will be enough time to get the patient to a nearby hospital. Contractions less than 2 minutes apart, especially in a multiparous woman (a woman who has had more than one pregnancy, sometimes called a "multip" for short), signal impending delivery.
- Has the amniotic sac ruptured and, if so, when? If the sac ruptures more than 18 hours before birth occurs, the likelihood of fetal infection is increased, and the hospital staff should be alerted. Furthermore, delivery may be more difficult when the amniotic sac has ruptured prematurely, as amniotic fluid serves as a lubricant.
- Does the mother feel as though she has to move her bowels? This sensation is caused by the fetal head in the vagina pressing against the rectum and indicates that delivery is imminent.

The mother also should be examined to see whether the fetus is crowning. When crowning occurs, the vaginal opening will bulge outward and the presenting part of the fetus will be visible at the opening. Crowning indicates that the fetus is about to be born, and there will not be time to go to the hospital before delivery.

If there is enough time to transport the patient to the hospital, she should be placed in a reclining position during transport. Any underclothing that might obstruct delivery should be removed. The paramedic should:

- Never allow the mother to go to the toilet
- Never attempt to delay or restrain delivery in any way

If there is not enough time to get to the hospital, the paramedic must prepare to assist in delivery. If the mother is in a crowded or public place, the paramedic should try to find a private clean area in which to work. The patient may find it reassuring to have her husband or a friend present. Paramedics should remain calm, as this will exert a calming influence on the patient and any others present.

The patient should be positioned on her back, on the stretcher or in bed, and a folded sheet or drape should be placed under her buttocks. She then should bend her knees and spread her thighs apart. As soon as the paramedic and assistant finish positioning the mother, the assistant should start an IV with 1 1 of D5W to a keep open rate. The paramedic should go then to the mother's head and be prepared to turn her head to the side if she vomits. An oxygen tank and suction apparatus should be readily available.

Hands should be washed thoroughly before the obstetrical (OB) kit is opened. Betadine scrub solution should be kept with the kit for this purpose. The OB kit should be opened, and the paramedic should put on sterile gloves. The mother should be draped with four towels so that everything except the vaginal opening is thoroughly covered. If the baby is coming fast, it is more important for the paramedic to assist in the delivery than to put on drapes or gloves. The paramedic should encourage the mother to relax and to take slow, deep breaths through her mouth and should continue to reassure her and explain everything that is being done.

When the baby's head begins to emerge from the vagina, it should be supported gently to prevent explosive delivery. The paramedic should not attempt to pull the baby from the vagina. If the membranes cover the head after it emerges, the sac should be torn with fingers or forceps and removed from the infant's face to permit the amniotic fluid to escape so that the infant will be able to breathe. The paramedic must be sure the umbilical cord is not wrapped around the infant's neck; if it is, it should be slipped gently over the shoulder or head. If this maneuver fails and the cord is tight around the baby's neck, umbilical clamps should be placed rapidly on the cord 2 inches apart and the cord should be cut between the clamps to release pressure on the infant's neck. The shoulders and body should be delivered with the head supported at all times. The paramedic should avoid touching the mother's anus during delivery. The time of birth should be recorded.

After the baby is fully delivered, he or she should be supported along the length of the paramedic's arm, with one arm and shoulder supported by the paramedic's cupped fingers. The infant's head should be held downward to aid drainage. Babies must be held carefully, as they are slippery. Any blood and mucus from the nose and mouth should be wiped away with a piece of sterile gauze. The mouth and both nostrils should be suctioned with a bulb aspirator. The paramedic should squeeze the bulb before inserting the tip of the aspirator and then place the tip in the mouth or nostrils and release bulb slowly. The contents of the bulb can be expelled into a waste container, and suctioning can be repeated as needed.

If the baby does not breathe spontaneously, the paramedic should stimulate the infant by rubbing the back gently or slapping the soles of the feet. If there is still no response, the paramedic should start mouth-to-mouth or mouth-to-nose resuscitation, remembering that newborn infants are very little and thus require very small puffs of air. Mechanical resuscitation devices should never be used on a newborn infant. If spontaneous breathing begins, oxygen should be administered by mask for a few minutes, until the baby's color is pink. If breathing is still absent, however, and no precordial pulse can be determined with the stethoscope, cardiac compression should be started and cardiopulmonary resuscitation should be continued en route to the hospital. The baby should be kept wrapped in a blanket as much as possible.

If, however, the infant has been delivered normally and is breathing well, the cord should be clamped about 6 inches from the infant's navel with two clamps set 3 inches apart. If clamps are unavailable, two umbilical ties can be substituted. The cord should be cut between the two ties and handled gently because it will tear easily. The end of the cord that is attached to the infant must be examined to be certain there is no bleeding. If there is bleeding from a cut end, the cord proximal to the clamp should be tied and reexamined. The baby should then be wrapped in a sterile blanket to maintain body temperature.

During the next stage of delivery, one paramedic should stand at the mother's head and keep an eye on the infant, while the other paramedic tends to the delivery of the placenta. The placenta usually is delivered spontaneously within 15 to 20 minutes after the infant's birth. Bleeding can be expected as the placenta separates from the uterine wall. When bleeding occurs, the uterus should be gently massaged. Uterine massage will stimulate the uterus to contract, thus constricting blood vessels within its walls and decreasing bleeding. Allowing the infant to nurse following the delivery of the placenta will control bleeding as nursing stimulates the release of oxytocin. Oxytocin, in addition to causing milk ejection, stimulates uterine contraction, which constricts uterine blood vessels.

The paramedic should never pull on the umbilical cord to deliver the placenta. Pulling can invert the uterus (cause it to turn inside out). When the placenta is delivered, it should be placed in a basin or plastic bag and taken to the hospital, where it will be examined for completeness. This procedure is necessary because pieces of placenta retained in the uterus cause persistent bleeding. The perineum, the skin between the anus and the vagina, should be examined for lacerations, and pressure applied to any bleeding tears with a sanitary napkin. 'A sanitary napkin then should be placed over the vagina, the mother's legs can be lowered, and she can be prepared for transport to the hospital. If the physician orders it, the mother can be given 10 units of oxytocin (Pitocin) slowly IV.

If the placenta is not delivered within about 15 to 20 minutes after the baby's delivery, the mother and baby should be transported to the hospital without further delay.

Complications of Delivery

Three types of problems that can accompany delivery will be discussed in this section: postpartum hemorrhage, uterine inversion, and pulmonary embolism. The paramedic should be prepared to treat each of these situations as it occurs.

Postpartum hemorrhage. Postpartum hemorrhage occurs after delivery and is characterized by internal or external bleeding.

Internal bleeding.--Internal bleeding may be caused by retained placental tissue, inadequate uterine contractions, or clotting disorders. If bleeding is severe, uterine massage should be continued, and the baby should be allowed to suckle the mother's breast. The paramedic can add 10 units of oxytocin to the IV bottle following delivery of the placenta. If bleeding persists, the circulation can be supported with an IV of normal saline, Ringer's solution, or plasma derivative. The patient should be transported rapidly to the hospital, and the usual measures for shock should be applied. Vaginal examination or blind packing of the vagina should be avoided. Gentle uterine massage should be continued en route to the hospital.

External bleeding.--External bleeding from perineal tears can be managed with firm pressure. It may be necessary to open the labia to apply packs to the bleeding site.

Uterine inversion. Inversion, or turning inside out, of the uterus can occur as a result of excessive pressure on the uterus or from pulling on the umbilical cord in efforts to deliver the placenta. Shock commonly accompanies uterine inversion. Should this condition occur in the field, the paramedic should take the following steps:

- Keep patient flat.
- Administer oxygen.
- Start two IV lines with Ringer's solution or colloid, running them as fast as necessary to maintain blood pressure.
- Never try to remove the placenta if it is still attached.
- Try once to replace the uterus manually by exerting pressure first on the area closest to the cervix. If. the uterus cannot be replaced easily, pack all protruding tissues lightly with moist, sterile towels, and move the patient rapidly to the hospital.

Pulmonary embolism. Sudden dyspnea, tachypnea, tachycardia, and/or hypotension in the mother post partum can signal pulmonary embolism, either from a blood clot or from amniotic fluid. Field treatment is the same as for any patient with pulmonary embolism and includes administration of oxygen, electrocardiogram monitoring, and rapid transport to the hospital.

Abnormal Deliveries

Deliveries in which the fetal head does not present first are classified as abnormal deliveries. Three abnormal presentations will be discussed in this section: breech presentation, prolapsed umbilical cord, and limb presentation. These three situations can be potentially life threatening to the infant, and thus the paramedic should become familiar with the special problems of each situation.

Breech presentation. Breech presentation occurs when the buttocks rather than the head present first. Breech delivery is not a simple delivery. If delivery is imminent, the mother should be prepared as discussed earlier, and the buttocks and trunk of the baby should be allowed to deliver spontaneously. Once the legs are clear, the baby's body should be supported on the palm of the paramedic's hand and the anterior surface of the paramedic's arm, thus allowing the head to deliver. If the head is not delivered within 3 minutes, action must be taken to prevent suffocation of the infant. Suffocation can occur when the baby's face is pressed against the vaginal wall or when the umbilical cord is compressed by the baby's head in the vagina. To establish an airway in the first instance, the paramedic should:

- Place a gloved hand in the vagina, positioning the palm toward the baby's face
- Form a "V" with the fingers on either side of the baby's nose
- Push the vaginal wall away from the baby's face until the head is delivered

To relieve pressure on the umbilical cord, the paramedic can use one of the following techniques:

- Place the patient in a supine (Trendelenburg) position, and apply gentle pressure to the buttocks, forcing the baby back into the uterus and out of the vagina.
- Place a gloved hand inside the vagina with fingers separated, allowing the cord to pass through the opening created by the fingers between the cervical side wall and the baby's head.

The paramedic should neither try to pull the baby out of the vagina nor allow explosive delivery. If the head does not deliver within 3 minutes after an airway has been established, the mother should be placed in Trendelenburg position and be transported rapidly to the hospital. The baby's airway should be maintained throughout transport.

Prolapsed umbilical cord. Prolapsed umbilical cord occurs when the cord comes out of the vagina before the baby. The baby is, therefore, in danger of suffocation because the cord is compressed against the birth canal by the baby's head and the supply of oxygenated blood from the placenta is cut off. Rapid treatment is essential. To prevent the baby's suffocation, the paramedic should:

- Place the mother supine or on her side (in Trendelenberg position) with her hips elevated on a pillow, and make sure she is kept warm
- Administer oxygen to the mother
- With a gloved hand, gently push the baby back up into the vagina several inches
- Never attempt to push the cord back
- Transport the mother and the baby to the hospital at once, while maintaining pressure on the baby's head (pressure should be evenly distributed to avoid injury to the baby's soft skull)

Breech presentation and prolapsed umbilical cord are the only two cases in which the paramedic should place his or her hand in the mother's vagina.

Limb presentation. The presentation of an arm or leg through the vagina is an indication for immediate transport to the hospital, the only place where such a delivery should be attempted.

Other Childbirth Situations

Other unusual childbirth situations that the paramedic may encounter include multiple and premature births. These are of concern primarily because premature infants, and occasionally multiple-birth infants, require special care because of their small size.

Multiple births. Multiple births usually do not present any unique problems. Twins are delivered in the same manner as single babies. Twins should be anticipated if the mother's abdomen appears unusually large or if it remains large after the (first) baby is delivered. If twins are expected, the mother should be transported to the hospital as quickly as possible. After the first baby is born, the cord should be tied off to prevent hemorrhage from the twin. If the second baby is not delivered within 10 minutes of the first, the mother should be transported to the hospital for delivery of the second twin. Twins tend to be small and, like premature infants, need special protection against fall in body temperature. It is essential that twins be kept warm during transport.

Premature births. Any baby born before 7 months of pregnancy or weighing less than 2,500 grams (g) (5.5 pounds) is defined as premature and needs special care. Birth weight alone is not an adequate definition for prematurity because low-birth-weight infants may be fully mature. Conversely, premature infants may be over 2,500 g if they are edematous or if their mothers are diabetic. To distinguish premature from mature infants, the paramedic should observe the creases on the soles of their feet, breast size, type of scalp hair, and presence or absence of cartilage in their outer ears. Infants of less than 36-weeks (8-months) gestation have a single anterior sole crease; breast nodules that are 2 millimeters (mm) or less in diameter; fine, fuzzy scalp hair; and absent external ear cartilage. The heads of premature infants are also larger in proportion to their bodies than those of full-term infants. Infants of at least 39-weeks gestation have creases covering the soles of their feet; breast nodules 7 or more in diameter; coarse, silky scalp hair; and cartilaginous outer ears.

Premature infants develop problems both because they are so small and because their organs are immature. Premature infants have trouble maintaining a normal body temperature because they have more surface area relative to their size than older people and, therefore, lose heat more rapidly in a cool environment. In addition, premature babies have less subcutaneous fat to insulate them against heat loss.

Small blood losses are also more serious in premature infants because of their small size. The 2,500-g infant has a total blood volume of about 275 milliliters (ml). Therefore, 30-ml blood loss represents 10 percent of the infant's total blood volume.

Premature infants often develop respiratory problems because their lungs are immature. Alveoli and alveolar capillaries begin developing at 28-weeks gestation. Surfactant, which lowers alveolar surface tension and allows even expansion of the alveoli, similarly develops at about 28-weeks gestation.

Hypoxemia due to respiratory problems leads to cardiovascular problems in the premature infant. Before birth, blood is shunted past the lungs and oxygenated in the placenta. After birth, special mechanisms change the blood flow pattern, so that blood is oxygenated in the lungs. These special mechanisms, however, depend on adequate oxygenation of the blood by the lungs. When oxygenation is inadequate due to lung immaturity, blood continues to be shunted past the lungs. This worsens the hypoxemia. Hypoxemia due to respiratory and cardiovascular problems produces cyanosis and leads to bradycardia (in the newborn infant, bradycardia is a heart rate less than 100) and hypotension.

The premature infant also tolerates asphyxia normally occurring during labor and delivery less well than the full-term infant. The mature infant survives some asphyxia during labor and delivery by metabolizing liver and heart glycogen stores. The premature infant, however, has less stored glycogen and, therefore, is less able to tolerate asphyxia.

To manage the premature infant the paramedic should:

- Keep the baby warm. Wrap the baby in aluminum foil and blankets to reduce heat loss.
- Keep the baby's nose and mouth clear of fluid with a bulb syringe.
- Prevent bleeding from the umbilical cord as these infants cannot tolerate the loss of even small amounts of blood.
- Give oxygen into a tent constructed from aluminum foil above the infant's head. Do not blast it directly into the infant's face.
- Prevent contamination as premature infants are highly susceptible to infection.

Apgar Scoring

It is important for the newborn to be evaluated immediately after birth to determine adequacy of vital functions. The scoring system devised by Virginia Apgar is helpful in this evaluation. It is based on heart rate, respiratory effort, muscle tone, reflex irritability, and color. Sixty seconds after the birth of the infant, these five signs are evaluated and each given a score of 0, 1, or 2. When added together, numerical ratings yielding a total score of 10 indicate that the infant is in excellent condition. The majority of infants are vigorous and have a total score of 7 to 10; they cough or cry within seconds of delivery and require no further resuscitation. Infants with a score in the 4 to 6 range are moderately depressed. They may be pale or blue 1 minute after delivery, with poorly sustained respiration and flaccid muscle tone. Such infants will require some form of resuscitation.

The five signs to be evaluated in Apgar scoring are most easily remembered by using the mnemonic APGAR, as shown in Table 11.1.

TABLE 11.1
Apgar Score

Sign	Score 0	Score 1	Score 2
A--Appearance (color)	Absent	Slow or less than 100	Greater than 100
P--Pulse (heart rate)	Absent	Slow, irregular	Good; crying
G--Grimace (reflex irritability)	Limp	Some flexion of extremities	Active motion
A--Activity (muscle tone)	No response	Grimace	Cough or sneeze
R--Respiration (respiratory effort)	Blue, pale	Body pink; extremities blue	Completely pink

GLOSSARY

abortion: Premature expulsion of the products of conception from the uterus; abortion can occur naturally or can be artificially induced.

incomplete abortion: When part of the fetus or parts of the products of conception are expelled; when parts of the products of conception are expelled from the uterus and parts remain inside.

inevitable abortion: An abortion that cannot be halted; characterized by vaginal bleeding, uterine contractions and cervical dilation before term. missed abortion: An abortion when the fetus dies before 20-weeks gestation but is retained in the uterus for 2 months following death.

spontaneous abortion: An abortion occurring naturally.

therapeutic abortion: A legal, induced abortion performed under sterile conditions in an authorized medical setting. threatened abortion: The appearance of signs and symptoms of possible loss of the fetus; characterized by bleeding and cramps.

abruptio placentae: A premature separation of a normally implanted placenta from the uterine wall, usually occurring during the third trimester of pregnancy and accompanied by pain and hemorrhage.

amniotic fluid: The fluid that surrounds the fetus in the uterus; contained in the amniotic sac.

amniotic sac: A thin, transparent sac that holds the fetus suspended in amniotic fluid.

Apgar score: A method, developed by Virginia Apgar, of assessing the newborn by designation of a score between o and 2 for the infant's appearance (color), pulse (heart rate), grimace (reflex irritability), activity (muscle tone) , and respiration (respiratory effort) at 1 minute after birth.

breech delivery: A delivery in which the presenting part of the fetus is the buttocks or foot instead of the head.

cephalic delivery: A delivery in which the fetus emerges head first; generally considered the normal mode of delivery.

cervix: The lower portion, or neck, of the uterus.

crowning: The stage of birth when the presenting part of the fetus is visible at the vaginal orifice.

eclampsia: A toxic condition that can occur during pregnancy; characterized by hypertension, edema, proteinuria, and seizures.

fallopian tube: The tube extending from an ovary to the uterus.

fetus: An unborn child after the 2d month of pregnancy.

labor: The muscular contractions of the uterus designed to expel the fetus from the mother.

limb presentation: A delivery in which the presenting part of a fetus is an arm or a leg.

menstrual period: The time period of the menstrual flow, usually from 3 to 7 days.

ovary: The female sex organ in which eggs and female hormones are produced.

ovum: An egg; plural form is ova.

perineum: The region of the body into which the urethral, vaginal, and rectal orifices open.

placenta: A vascular organ attached to the uterine wall that supplies oxygen and nutrients to the fetus; also called the afterbirth.

placenta previa: A delivery in which the placenta is the presenting part; may result in exsanguinating hemorrhage.

preeclampsia: The condition that precedes eclampsia, or toxemia of pregnancy; characterized by hypertension and edema.

presenting part: The part of the fetus that emerges first during delivery.

prolapsed cord: A delivery in which the umbilical cord is the presenting part; fetal suffocation is a danger in this delivery.

toxemia: A condition sometimes occurring during the second half of pregnancy, manifested by symptoms of eclampsia.

vagina: The genital canal in the female extending from the uterus to the vulva; the birth canal.

ANSWER SHEET

TEST NO. ______________ PART ______ TITLE OF POSITION ______________________________
(AS GIVEN IN EXAMINATION ANNOUNCEMENT - INCLUDE OPTION, IF ANY)

PLACE OF EXAMINATION ______________________________ (CITY OR TOWN) ______________ (STATE) DATE ______________

RATING

USE THE SPECIAL PENCIL. MAKE GLOSSY BLACK MARKS.

1 A B C D E	26 A B C D E	51 A B C D E	76 A B C D E	101 A B C D E
2 A B C D E	27 A B C D E	52 A B C D E	77 A B C D E	102 A B C D E
3 A B C D E	28 A B C D E	53 A B C D E	78 A B C D E	103 A B C D E
4 A B C D E	29 A B C D E	54 A B C D E	79 A B C D E	104 A B C D E
5 A B C D E	30 A B C D E	55 A B C D E	80 A B C D E	105 A B C D E
6 A B C D E	31 A B C D E	56 A B C D E	81 A B C D E	106 A B C D E
7 A B C D E	32 A B C D E	57 A B C D E	82 A B C D E	107 A B C D E
8 A B C D E	33 A B C D E	58 A B C D E	83 A B C D E	108 A B C D E
9 A B C D E	34 A B C D E	59 A B C D E	84 A B C D E	109 A B C D E
10 A B C D E	35 A B C D E	60 A B C D E	85 A B C D E	110 A B C D E

Make only ONE mark for each answer. Additional and stray marks may be counted as mistakes. In making corrections, erase errors COMPLETELY.

11 A B C D E	36 A B C D E	61 A B C D E	86 A B C D E	111 A B C D E
12 A B C D E	37 A B C D E	62 A B C D E	87 A B C D E	112 A B C D E
13 A B C D E	38 A B C D E	63 A B C D E	88 A B C D E	113 A B C D E
14 A B C D E	39 A B C D E	64 A B C D E	89 A B C D E	114 A B C D E
15 A B C D E	40 A B C D E	65 A B C D E	90 A B C D E	115 A B C D E
16 A B C D E	41 A B C D E	66 A B C D E	91 A B C D E	116 A B C D E
17 A B C D E	42 A B C D E	67 A B C D E	92 A B C D E	117 A B C D E
18 A B C D E	43 A B C D E	68 A B C D E	93 A B C D E	118 A B C D E
19 A B C D E	44 A B C D E	69 A B C D E	94 A B C D E	119 A B C D E
20 A B C D E	45 A B C D E	70 A B C D E	95 A B C D E	120 A B C D E
21 A B C D E	46 A B C D E	71 A B C D E	96 A B C D E	121 A B C D E
22 A B C D E	47 A B C D E	72 A B C D E	97 A B C D E	122 A B C D E
23 A B C D E	48 A B C D E	73 A B C D E	98 A B C D E	123 A B C D E
24 A B C D E	49 A B C D E	74 A B C D E	99 A B C D E	124 A B C D E
25 A B C D E	50 A B C D E	75 A B C D E	100 A B C D E	125 A B C D E

ANSWER SHEET

TEST NO. ______________ PART ______ TITLE OF POSITION ______________________________

(AS GIVEN IN EXAMINATION ANNOUNCEMENT - INCLUDE OPTION, IF ANY)

PLACE OF EXAMINATION ______________________________ ______________ DATE ______________

(CITY OR TOWN) (STATE)

RATING

USE THE SPECIAL PENCIL. MAKE GLOSSY BLACK MARKS.

No.	A B C D E	No.	A B C D E	No.	A B C D E	No.	A B C D E	No.	A B C D E
1	A B C D E	26	A B C D E	51	A B C D E	76	A B C D E	101	A B C D E
2	A B C D E	27	A B C D E	52	A B C D E	77	A B C D E	102	A B C D E
3	A B C D E	28	A B C D E	53	A B C D E	78	A B C D E	103	A B C D E
4	A B C D E	29	A B C D E	54	A B C D E	79	A B C D E	104	A B C D E
5	A B C D E	30	A B C D E	55	A B C D E	80	A B C D E	105	A B C D E
6	A B C D E	31	A B C D E	56	A B C D E	81	A B C D E	106	A B C D E
7	A B C D E	32	A B C D E	57	A B C D E	82	A B C D E	107	A B C D E
8	A B C D E	33	A B C D E	58	A B C D E	83	A B C D E	108	A B C D E
9	A B C D E	34	A B C D E	59	A B C D E	84	A B C D E	109	A B C D E
10	A B C D E	35	A B C D E	60	A B C D E	85	A B C D E	110	A B C D E

Make only ONE mark for each answer. Additional and stray marks may be counted as mistakes. In making corrections, erase errors COMPLETELY.

No.	A B C D E	No.	A B C D E	No.	A B C D E	No.	A B C D E	No.	A B C D E
11	A B C D E	36	A B C D E	61	A B C D E	86	A B C D E	111	A B C D E
12	A B C D E	37	A B C D E	62	A B C D E	87	A B C D E	112	A B C D E
13	A B C D E	38	A B C D E	63	A B C D E	88	A B C D E	113	A B C D E
14	A B C D E	39	A B C D E	64	A B C D E	89	A B C D E	114	A B C D E
15	A B C D E	40	A B C D E	65	A B C D E	90	A B C D E	115	A B C D E
16	A B C D E	41	A B C D E	66	A B C D E	91	A B C D E	116	A B C D E
17	A B C D E	42	A B C D E	67	A B C D E	92	A B C D E	117	A B C D E
18	A B C D E	43	A B C D E	68	A B C D E	93	A B C D E	118	A B C D E
19	A B C D E	44	A B C D E	69	A B C D E	94	A B C D E	119	A B C D E
20	A B C D E	45	A B C D E	70	A B C D E	95	A B C D E	120	A B C D E
21	A B C D E	46	A B C D E	71	A B C D E	96	A B C D E	121	A B C D E
22	A B C D E	47	A B C D E	72	A B C D E	97	A B C D E	122	A B C D E
23	A B C D E	48	A B C D E	73	A B C D E	98	A B C D E	123	A B C D E
24	A B C D E	49	A B C D E	74	A B C D E	99	A B C D E	124	A B C D E
25	A B C D E	50	A B C D E	75	A B C D E	100	A B C D E	125	A B C D E